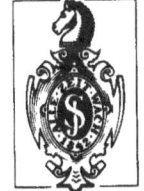

 The Bloomsbury Series in Clinical Science

BRONCHOALVEOLAR MAST CELLS AND ASTHMA

K. C. FLINT

with the assistance of B. N. Hudspith

With 29 Figures

Springer-Verlag
London Berlin Heidelberg New York
Paris Tokyo

✠ Kevin Charles Flint, BA, MB.BChir, MRCP

Barry Nicholson Hudspith, Chartered Biologist, MIBiol
Department of Immunology, The Middlesex Hospital Medical
School, London W1

Series Editor

Jack Tinker, BSc, FRCS, FRCP, DIC
Director, Intensive Therapy Unit, The Middlesex Hospital,
London W1N 8AA

Cover illustration: Scanning electron microscope photo of a
degranulating mast cell (reproduced by permission of Janssen
Pharmaceutica from their slide series "Allergy").

ISBN-13:978-1-4471-1460-4   e-ISBN-13:978-1-4471-1458-1
DOI: 10.1007/978-1-4471-1458-1

British Library Cataloguing in Publication Data
Flint, K. C.
Bronchoalveolar mast cells and asthma. ——
(The Bloomsbury series in clinical science).
1. Asthma   2. Mast cells
I. Title   II. Series
616.2'38   RC591
ISBN-13:978-1-4471-1460-4

This work is subject to copyright. All rights are reserved, whether the whole or part
of the material is concerned, specifically the rights of translation, reprinting, re-use
of illustrations, recitation, broadcasting, reproduction on microfilms or in other
ways, and storage in data banks. Duplication of this publication or parts thereof is
only permitted under the provisions of the German Copyright Law of September 9,
1965, in its version of June 24, 1985, and a copyright fee must always be paid.
Violations fall under the prosecution act of the German Copyright Law.

© Springer-Verlag Berlin Heidelberg 1987

The use of registered names, trademarks, etc. in this publication does not imply,
even in the absence of a specific statement, that such names are exempt from the
relevant protective laws and regulations and therefore free for general use.

Product Liability: The publisher can give no guarantee for information about drug
dosage and application thereof contained in this book. In every individual case the
respective user must check its accuracy by consulting other pharmaceutical
literature.

Filmset by Wilmaset, Birkenhead, Wirral.

For Marion, Lucy, Sam and Elizabeth

Tragically, Kevin Flint was killed, having prepared the first draft of the manuscript for this book. Barry Hudspith has put many hours into the re-writing and editing of the original script and the preparation of the illustrations in order that the final book could be published as a tribute to the work that Kevin and Barry performed together in our laboratories.

N.McI.J.

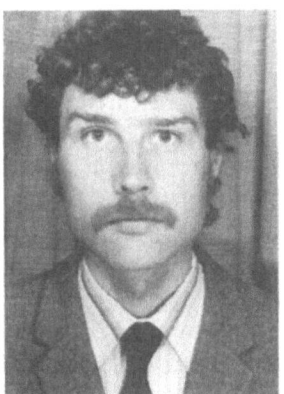

Kevin Charles Flint, BA, MB.BChir, MRCP
(20th Sept. 1952 – 20th Jan. 1986)

Kevin Charles Flint, Sir Jules Thorn Research Fellow to the Medical Unit of The Middlesex Hospital, was killed in tragic circumstances in a "hit and run" motor accident on 20th January 1986.

He was educated at the City of Leicester Boys' School and St. Catharine's College, Cambridge, where he took a BA in Physiology before reading Medicine. He completed his clinical training at the Middlesex Hospital Medical School, qualifying in 1978. After preregistration posts in St. Albans, he spent a year as Senior House Officer in Medicine at the Lister Hospital, Stevenage, followed by a year as Registrar in St. Albans, during which time he gained his MRCP. For the last 4 years he worked at the Middlesex Hospital, first as Registrar to the Professorial Medical Unit and finally as Sir Jules Thorn Research Fellow.

He was a young man of outstanding ability and promise. Throughout his medical training he had shown himself to be an extremely enthusiastic and excellent physician who was highly regarded and liked by his colleagues and patients. He was totally committed to The Middlesex and there was never anything he considered too much effort; such thoughts were foreign to a person with his drive and vitality. His chosen speciality was Respiratory Medicine and during his Research Fellowship he performed fundamental studies into the pathophysiology of asthma. He was one of the first people to recognise the possible role of the bronchoalveolar mast cell in this condition. Not only did he enumerate these cells and discover the differences found in asthma, he also developed a model for functional studies on these cells which may prove highly relevant for the in vitro assessment of new asthma therapies. His research work yielded 32 publications in the last 2 years, on 21 of which he was the first author. In 1984 he was awarded the Medical Research Society Essay Prize and his MD Thesis was submitted to Cambridge University a fortnight before his death. He had contributed chapters to books on asthma and sarcoidosis and was in the process of completing this monograph on the mast cell.

He presented his research frequently at both the Medical Research and British Thoracic Societies. In addition, in the last year he had given invited lectures both in the United States and Europe. He was an enthusiastic teacher both of undergraduates and postgraduates and was in great demand, both for his lecturing and bedside teaching.

He had been "head hunted" for a fulltime career in research on more than one occasion. However, his commitment to the National Health Service as a concept and his love of clinical medicine made him decline these offers. He preferred to seek promotion within the conventional channels and was to be promoted to Lecturer within a few days of his death. His ultimate ambition was to become a teaching hospital Consultant Physician – none of those who knew him doubted that this was likely within a few years.

He was a kind, considerate and unassuming physician who will be missed by all his colleagues and patients, to all of whom he was regarded as a friend above all else. He had a lively sense of humour and total commitment to life, both at work and at home with his young family to whom he was absolutely devoted. He is survived by his wife Marion, his daughter Lucy, his son Sam and Elizabeth, their 3-month-old baby.

N. McI. J.

Reproduced by the kind permission of the *British Medical Journal*.

Series Editor's Foreword

The publication of *Bronchoalveolar Mast Cells and Asthma* marks the emergence of The Bloomsbury Series in Clinical Science, an important and novel series that will highlight, review and record major areas of research, development and practice in the field of clinical science. A number of other monographs are now in an advanced state of preparation and their release will establish not only their individual significance but that of the series as a whole.

My thanks are due to the Editorial Board who have provided the ideas and selected the authors and whose continuing enthusiasm is so vital to the success of the series. Michael Jackson of Springer-Verlag merits special thanks for initially realising the potential of such a series and then guiding us all through to the time of its launch. Marianne Williams has supported us all and has provided the important link between Editorial Board and publisher.

The author of this first publication, Kevin Flint, was tragically killed during its preparation, and we hope that the book will serve as a tribute to the memory of Kevin for all who were lucky enough to know him. Barry Hudspith has been of enormous help in finalising the work and in shaping the form of the book.

Bronchoalveolar Mast Cells and Asthma is based on the work Kevin Flint did for his MD thesis. It gives a clear insight into the role of mast cells and their relation to asthma via a host of mediators. An understanding of these provides the scientific basis for the modern management of the asthmatic patient.

London, August 1987   Jack Tinker

Preface

It has been demonstrated that the technique of bronchoalveolar lavage offers the opportunity to study the function of cells of the human mucosal immune system in vitro. Kevin Flint suggested that mast cells found within this population of cells would be situated in an ideal position to mediate the cascade of reactions that lead to the condition known as asthma. This is because antigen challenge in by far the majority of cases will occur via the airways. Lying superficially within these airways, bronchoalveolar mast cells would be in an ideal position to interact with inhaled antigen and mediators released by bronchoalveolar mast cells would be released directly into the airway surface. Bronchoalveolar mast cells would therefore be ideally placed to mediate the rapid bronchial reactions which follow the inhalation of allergen in asthmatic subjects. Bronchoalveolar mast cells have several other advantages over the dispersed human lung mast cell preparation. They are not subjected to mechanical or enzymic trauma, being obtained by simple saline lavage. They are therefore more likely to respond in vitro in a manner resembling their response in vivo. Perhaps their greatest advantage is that bronchoalveolar mast cells can be obtained from subjects with widely differing underlying pathologies. We therefore now have the opportunity to study the function of mast cells from different pathological situations.

For his M.D. research project, Dr Flint characterised the morphology of bronchoalveolar mast cells and showed that these cells could release histamine and other mediators in response to immunological challenge. He demonstrated that these responses could be inhibited by drugs known to act as anti-asthmatic agents. This work led him to the conclusion that bronchoalveolar lavage was a more appropriate model of lung mast cell function than the more traditionally used human dispersed lung cells for clinical research purposes both for studies into basic mechanisms of disease and for the screening of potentially clinically useful drugs.

Contents

The work of Dr Flint presented in this book establishes bronchoalveolar lavage as a useful in vitro model of human mast cell function and demonstrates its great potential for the study into the role of this cell in health and disease. He was a dedicated research worker and an enthusiastic teacher of his subject, and his work will form the basis of many further advances in this area of research in the next few years.

Acknowledgements

Kevin Flint wrote this book on the basis of the work he did at the Middlesex Hospital, London, for his MD thesis. Those he acknowledged for their support then were Dr. N. McI. Johnson for his help and guidance throughout this study, Dr. F. L. Pearce for his excellent advice, K. B. P. Leung for help with the in vitro experiments, Kaye Seager and Dr. M. Hammond of Miles Laboratories, Stoke Poges, for the measurements of leukotriene C_4 and prostaglandin D_2, and the Sir Jules Thorn Trust for financial support.

We would also like to acknowledge Dr. T. S. C. Orr and Dr. L. Bjermer of Fisons Pharmaceuticals, Loughborough, for the kind permission to publish the EM pictures of mast cells reproduced in Chapter 2 of this book, and Margot Tomlinson for typing the manuscript.

London, 1987

B. N. Hudspith

Chapter 1

Mast Cells and the Allergic Response

Introduction

The word asthma derives from the Greek ασθμα (meaning panting). It is a disease characterised by widespread and variable obstruction of the intrathoracic airways. Such a functional definition does not imply a specific cause or mechanism whether it be neurological, immunological or pharmacological. It is a multifactorial and protean disease with many distinct clinical forms which has so far defied any unifying hypothesis (Turner-Warwick 1978).

In recent years, it has become evident that the mast cell occupies a central position in the pathogenesis of asthma. The evidence for this is considerable. Mast cells are widely distributed in the human body; they are especially prevalent at sites that come into contact with the external environment such as the skin, lung, nasal mucosa and gastrointestinal tract (Pepys and Edwards 1979), and can migrate to such sites during allergen exposure (Enerbäck et al. 1986). They are therefore ideally placed to play a fundamental role in allergic disorders.

Mast cells possess and can synthesise a wide range of pharmacologically active mediators which can be released after IgE-dependent mast cell activation in a rapid process that parallels the speed of immunological type I (immediate) allergic reactions in vivo. A host of inflammatory mediators are released, many being extremely potent substances having biological effects in minute quantities. However, clinical asthma is not only a rapid and transient process. In many subjects the early phase of bronchial obstruction after antigen challenge is followed by a later, sustained phase at 4–6 h (Warner 1978). This late phase reaction more closely resembles the clinical course of chronic asthma.

The pathological changes associated with asthma have been described in necropsy studies, both for patients dying during acute asthma attacks (Houston et al. 1953; Dunnill 1960; Salvato 1968) and after incidental deaths in asthmatic subjects (Dunnill 1965). Pathological changes are present throughout the lungs and persist even in remission (Dunnill 1965; Cutz et al. 1978). The most striking feature of the lungs at necropsy is their gross over-distension. Areas of collapse are sharply defined and the cut surface shows numerous glistening plugs of exudate in both small and large air passages (Dunnill 1965). The exudate consists of layers of mucus, inflammatory cells and epithelium which in these fatal cases may be shed over almost the entire airway surface (Lopez-Vidriero and Reid 1983). Mucus glands are often enlarged with increased numbers of goblet cells (Houston et al. 1953) and there is hypertrophy and hyperplasia of bronchial smooth muscle (Hossain 1973). The basement membrane thickening is typical (Dunnill 1965). A characteristic feature of asthma is the intense inflammatory infiltrate in the airway mucosa and air spaces. This consists mainly of eosinophils, with some neutrophils and mononuclear cells (Dunnill 1960, 1965; Cutz et al. 1978; Dunnill et al. 1969).

If the mast cell is to maintain its putative central role in asthma, mast cell activation must be shown to be capable of initiating the events which lead to the sustained bronchial obstruction and persistent inflammation seen in the clinical disease.

The hypothesis that mast cells have a role in asthma is outlined in Fig. 1.1. Antigen stimulation of an asthmatic attack will occur via the airways. Bronchoalveolar mast cells found lying superficially within these airways would be in an ideal position to interact with inhaled antigen and the mediators released by these cells would be released directly on to the airway surface. These bronchoalveolar mast cells would therefore be ideally placed to mediate the rapid bronchial reactions which would follow the inhalation of an allergen in an asthmatic subject. As it is the bronchoalveolar cell that is active in asthmatic

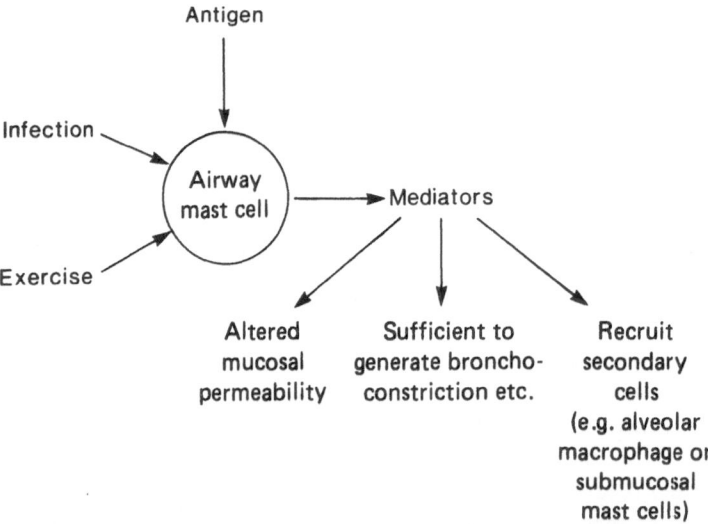

Fig. 1.1.   The proposed hypothesis of the central role of mast cells in asthma.

disease, I suggest that it is the mast cell recovered by bronchoalveolar lavage which should be studied, rather than the mast cell recovered from dispersed human lung.

Mast Cell Activation and Mediator Release

Mast Cell Activation

Many of the cellular events which accompany mast cell activation have now been identified. Mast cells possess high affinity membrane receptors for immunoglobulin E (IgE) (Tigelaar et al. 1971). The binding of divalent or multivalent antigen to receptor bound IgE, or the crosslinking of IgE by antibody to its Fc portion (anti-IgE antibody), results in mast cell activation (Levine and Fellner 1965; Ishizaka et al. 1971). The requirement for receptor bridging for mediator release is absolute, as demonstrated by the failure of Fab monomers of either anti-IgE or anti-IgE receptor antibodies to effect release (Ishizaka 1982). Cell activation–secretion is an energy dependent process and requires the activity of a diisopropyl fluorophosphonate (DFP)-sensitive serine esterase (Austen and Brocklehurst 1960; Ishizaka 1981). Two apparently concurrent transient events occur within 15 s of IgE receptor dimerisation: a rapid and transient rise in cyclic adenosine monophosphate (cyclic AMP) and phospholipid methylation. Hirata and Axelrod (1978) have identified two methyl transferases in the plasma membrane, one facing the cytoplasmic side and one the outer surface of the membrane. Following activation of rat mast cells by concanavalin A (Hirata et al. 1979) or IgE receptor perturbation (Ishizaka et al. 1980), phosphatidyl ethanolamine is methylated in the presence of S-adenosyl-methionine to phosphatidyl-n-monomethanolamine and then to phosphatidyl choline and translocated from the cytoplasmic to the extracellular side of the membrane. This reorientation of phospholipids increases membrane fluidity, which allows coupling of IgE-Fc receptors to adenylate cyclase and an increase in calcium flux through calcium channels into the cell (Ishizaka 1981). Inhibition of phospholipid methylation results in a dose-dependent inhibition of the initial rise in cyclic AMP, of calcium influx into the cell and of subsequent histamine release (Ishizaka et al. 1981; Ishizaka 1982). Calcium influx is probably linked with the intracellular calcium receptor, calmodulin, a protein which plays a regulatory role in the catalytic expression of a number of enzymes. A calcium–magnesium activated adenosine triphosphatase (ATPase) has been identified histochemically on the outer surface of rat peritoneal mast cells and granule membranes. This enzyme may provide energy for the contraction of the cytoskeletal elements that transport granules to the plasma membrane in preparation for fusion and secretion (Chakraverty 1980).

Transmembrane activation of adenylate cyclase generates cyclic AMP, which acts as a second messenger by activating cyclic AMP dependent protein kinases (Holgate et al. 1980). Activation of 95% pure rat serosal mast cells results in a monophasic rise in cyclic AMP reaching a maximum at 15 s and a second monophasic rise reaching a maximum between 2 and 5 min (Ishizaka 1981). A similar sequence of events has been identified following activation of dispersed human lung mast cells purified by countercurrent centrifugal elutriation and density gradient centrifugation although biochemical events appear to occur more slowly in the human mast cell system (Ishizaka 1984). Indomethacin abolishes the second rise but does not affect either the initial increase in cyclic AMP or histamine release (Lewis et al. 1979). Prostaglandin D_2 will elevate intracellular cyclic AMP and is also without effect on mediator release but elevation of cyclic AMP by beta receptor agonists leads to inhibition of mediator release (Marquardt and Wasserman 1982; Holgate et al. 1980; Peters et al. 1984). Further investigation has led to the concept of distinct intracellular pools of cyclic AMP, similar to those proposed for polymorphonuclear leucocytes (Earp and Steiner 1978). Thus, in the mast cell three different stimuli may result in elevation of cyclic AMP, each with different consequences (Holgate et al. 1980; Winslow and Austen 1982). Firstly, the early IgE–Fc receptor initiated rise in cyclic AMP associated with activation–secretion coupling. Secondly, the later, cyclooxygenase-dependent rise in cyclic AMP which is reproduced by prostaglandin D_2 but has no effect on mediator release. Thirdly, beta receptor agonist or methyl xanthine induced elevations of cyclic AMP which result in the inhibition of secretion.

The morphometric associations of activation–secretion have also been studied. Activation of mast cells leads to granule swelling and solubilisation of the matrix which is particularly well seen in human pulmonary mast cells (Caulfield et al. 1980). Following IgE-dependent activation the crystalline structure of the granule is lost and there is alignment of intermediate filaments around the perigranular membrane prior to movement towards and finally fusion with the plasma membrane. Release of preformed granule constituents occurs simultaneously with newly generated lipid materials and together these comprise the mediators of immediate hypersensitivity.

Mast Cell Mediators

Preformed Mediators

The preformed mediators of mast cells are stored within the granules or make up the matrix material of these granules. They include low molecular weight mediators, enzymes and chemotactic factors (Table 1.1). Of the mediators identified following the IgE-dependent activation of tissues, histamine is the one most closely associated with the mast cell. This vasoactive amine is formed by the action of the cytoplasmic enzyme histidine decarboxylase on the precursor histidine. It is stored bound to the protein and proteoglycan matrix of the mast cell granule (Lagunoff 1974; Uvnas and Aborg 1977) and released when exposed to the external environment after exocytosis (Uvnas et al. 1970). The actions of histamine, via both H_1 and H_2 receptors have been extensively investigated. H_1 receptor activation causes constriction of bronchial smooth muscle in vitro (Drazen and Schneider 1978) and in vivo (Loring et al. 1977; Woenne et al. 1978), increased vascular permeability (Pietro and Magno 1978), and mucus secretion in bronchial mucosal explants (Shelhamer et al. 1980). H_2 activation leads to an increased airway permeability to large molecules (Boucher et al. 1978; Braude et al. 1984) and it also promotes neutrophil and eosinophil chemotaxis and modulates lymphocyte function (Plaut et al. 1973; Rocklin and Haberek-Davidson 1981).

Table 1.1.   Granule stored mast cell mediators

Histamine	– Constricts bronchial smooth muscle [H_1] – Increases vascular permeability [H_1] – Increases airway permeability [H_2] – Increases mucus secretion [H_1] – Modulates neutrophils eosinophil and lymphocyte function
Heparin	– Proteoglycan matrix binding histamine – Combines with platelet factor IV – Anti-thrombin III
Neutral protease (tryptase)	– Cleaves complement component C3 – Cleaves high mol. wt. kininogen
β-Hexosaminadase Acid hydrolase Aryl sulphatase	? Potential inflammatory response
Inflammatory factors of anaphylaxis (IFAs)	– Persistent inflammatory cellular infiltrate
Eosinophil chemotactic factor of anaphylaxis (ECF-A)	– Eosinophil chemotaxis – Increase eosinophil C3b and C4 receptors
Neutrophil chemotactic factor (NCF—? mast cell derived)	– Neutrophil chemotaxis

The intense inflammatory infiltrate seen in asthma has stimulated a search for other chemotactic factors and a variety of chemotactic activities have been identified in association with the mast cell granule. Eosinophils in particular form a characteristic component of the inflammatory cell infiltrate of asthmatic airways (Dunnill et al. 1969). Anaphylactic challenge of passively sensitised human and guinea pig lung fragments releases a number of small acidic peptides (mol. wt. 300–3000) which preferentially attract eosinophils from a mixed leucocyte population (Kay and Austen 1971). This activity has been called eosinophil chemotactic factor of anaphylaxis (ECF–A). Two tetrapeptides with similar activity have been purified from extracts of whole lung tissue (Goetzl and Austen 1975). In addition to chemotaxis, ECF–A will increase the number and function of human eosinophil C3b and C4 receptors (Anwar and Kay 1977). A family of preformed high molecular weight eosinophilotactic materials have also been identified in the granules of rat mast cells (Boswell et al. 1978).

Neutrophils are also present in significant numbers in the inflammatory infiltrate of asthma. A neutrophil chemotactic activity (NCA) has been identified in the circulation of asthmatic patients after antigen (Atkins et al. 1977) or exercise challenge (Lee et al. 1982). Its mast cell origin has yet to be demonstrated conclusively, but the time course of release parallels that of histamine and its appearance is blocked by prior administration of sodium cromoglycate (Atkins et al. 1978). Release of NCA from human lung fragments has also been documented (O'Driscoll et al. 1983).

The presence of a late phase reaction following type I allergic reactions in vivo may in part be explained by the release of inflammatory factors termed inflammatory factors of anaphylaxis (IFA) which cause a sustained inflammatory cellular infiltrate. Degranulation of rat cutaneous mast cells by anti-IgE or the polyamine 48/80 leads to an initial polymorphonuclear infiltrate followed by a mononuclear cell infiltrate persisting for up to 24 h. This sequence can be replicated by the injection of isolated mast cell granules (Tannenbaum et al. 1980). Two factors with similar activity (a high molecular weight and a low molecular weight factor) have been purified from the granule matrix (Oertel and Kaliner 1981; Kaliner and Lemanske 1984). The eosinophilic characteristic of human late phase reactions may reflect the inherent tissue eosinophilia of atopic subjects as eosinophilic infiltrates can be induced in these animals by rendering the animals eosinophilic by injection of sephadex beads.

Histochemical analysis and subcellular fractionation have identified several enzymes in association with the mast cell granule. Although their in vitro activity is well known their precise role in homeostasis and disease has yet to be determined. It is likely that they potentiate the inflammatory response after mast cell degranulation in vivo. The major protein component of human mast cell granules is a neutral protease (tryptase) which cleaves peptide and ester bonds on the carboxyl side of amino acids (Schwartz et al. 1981). It will cleave complement component C3 to fragments C3a and C3b with the anaphylatoxic activity (C3a) being further degraded by the same enzyme in the presence of heparin (Schwartz et al. 1983). Although it will cleave high molecular weight kininogen, this does not result in the appearance of kinin activity (Maier et al. 1983). Rat neutral proteases have chymotryptic rather than tryptic activity. Two immunologically distinct proteases have been identified in rat mast cells from different locations but a similar distinction has not yet been identified in other species. Mast cell granules also contain an acid hydrolase hexosaminadase and arylsulphatase (Schwartz et al. 1979; Schwartz et al. 1981; Schechter et al. 1983).

The final major constituent of the mast cell granule is the proteoglycan. This consists of a protein core with glycosaminoglycan side chains. In rat peritoneal and human dispersed lung mast cells the major proteoglycan is heparin (Metcalfe et al. 1979). Heparin has anti-thrombin III activity and it combines with platelet factor IV (McLaren et al. 1980). It may play a role in the local homeostasis of inflammatory reactions during tissue injury.

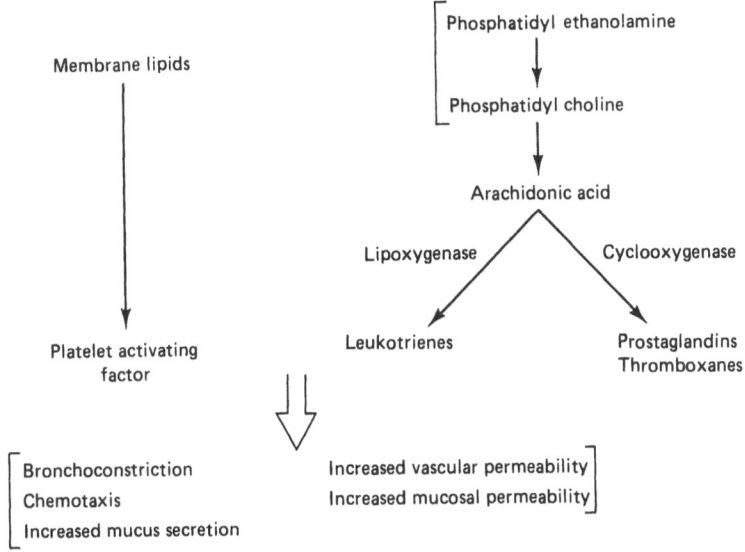

Fig. 1.2. Newly generated mediators of immediate hypersensitivity.

Newly Generated Mediators

Unstimulated mast cells do not contain all of the mediators detected after IgE-dependent mast cell activation; some are newly generated during the activation process (Fig. 1.2). The bridging of two or more mast cell surface IgE molecules activates a biochemical cascade beginning with the conversion of phosphatidyl ethanolamine to phosphatidyl choline. Arachidonic acid is largely although probably not exclusively derived from phosphatidyl choline by the action of a calcium dependent phospholipase A_2. The further metabolism of arachidonic acid occurs by two routes. The 5-lipoxygenase pathway leads to the sulphi-dopeptide leukotrienes, LTC_4, LTD_4 and LTE_4 now known to make up the major biological activity of slow reacting substance of anaphylaxis (SRS-A) (Morris et al. 1980; Bach et al. 1980). Arachidonic acid metabolism via the cyclooxygenase enzyme pathway leads to the generation of prostaglandins and thromboxanes.

A further major newly generated mediator is platelet activating factor (PAF). It is a phospholipid mediator originally identified by its ability to aggregate rabbit (Cazenave et al. 1979) and human platelets (Chignard et al. 1979). However, it is now apparent that it has a wide variety of other effects which may be relevant in the pathogenesis of asthma.

These three families of newly generated mediators are extremely potent biological substances having effects in minute quantities. These include bronchoconstriction, increased vascular permeability, increased mucus secretion and mucosal permeability and neutrophil and eosinophil chemotaxis. Many different cell types have the capacity to synthesise these mediators and their mast cell origin in allergic reactions has yet to be proven. A full discussion of this and the biological effects of newly generated mediators may be found in chapter 4.

Mast Cell Mediators and Their Antagonists In Vivo and In Vitro

Many attempts have been made to demonstrate the release of mast cell derived mediators in vivo during acute asthmatic reactions. Histamine has been identified in the sputum of asthmatic subjects (Turnbull et al. 1977; Bryant and Pui 1982) and the elevation of circulating plasma histamine found after antigen challenge supports the concept of mast cell activation in vivo (Brown et al. 1982). Classical H_1 receptor antagonists will inhibit the early phase of antigen-induced bronchial smooth muscle contraction in vitro (Adams and Lichtenstein 1979). Until recently it has proved difficult to demonstrate an effect of anti-histamines in vivo but with the development of better tolerated drugs an attenuation of both exercise and antigen-induced bronchoconstriction has now been demonstrated (Patel 1984; Hartley and Nogrady 1980). Antigen-induced contraction in vitro is only partially antagonised by concentrations of anti-histamine which will completely block the effect of exogenous histamine (Adams and Lichtenstein 1979) and attenuation of bronchoconstriction in vivo is incomplete, presumably because histamine is not the sole mediator of such reactions.

A rise in serum neutrophil chemotactic activities parallels increases in serum histamine during both early and late phase reactions following antigen or exercise provocation (Atkins et al. 1977; Atkins et al. 1978; Lee et al. 1982; Lee et al. 1984). The appearance of both can be blocked by sodium cromoglycate (Atkins et al. 1978). The precise cellular origin of NCA is undetermined but its release in IgE-dependent reactions in vitro is well documented (O'Driscoll et al. 1983).

The pharmaceutical industry has yet to develop a specific leukotriene antagonist sufficiently safe for use in human subjects. FPL 55712 was developed as an SRSA antagonist but its specificity of action is not certain. Adams and Lichtenstein (1979) found that while diphenhydramine (an H_1 antagonist) inhibited the early contractile response of passively sensitised human bronchial smooth muscle to ragweed antigen E, FPL 55712 inhibited the later phase of this response. Together these agents produced a dramatic attenuation of the response leaving a small residual contraction between 2 and 10 min. Although concentrations of FPL 55712 were high, with inevitable doubts about its specificity of action, this suggests a role for SRS-A in the sustained phase of bronchial smooth muscle contraction. Challenge with specific antigen results in contraction of bronchial smooth muscle obtained at postmortem from asthmatic subjects (Schild et al. 1951). Recently Hannsen et al. (1983) have shown release of leukotriene C_4, D_4 and E_4 simultaneous with a dose-dependent contraction of bronchial smooth muscle. Leukotriene release and smooth muscle contraction were both inhibited by a putative leukotriene inhibitor, U60257.

Identification of the newly generated mast cell mediators in vivo has proved difficult. An increase in the major metabolite of prostaglandin F_2alpha was found after antigen provocation (Green et al. 1974) but it is doubtful whether this prostaglandin is derived from lung mast cells. Leukotriene D_4 has been identified in the sputum of patients with cystic fibrosis (Cromwell et al. 1982) but not yet asthma and its measurement in serum is complicated by its rapid inactivation and protein binding (Morris et al. 1983).

Thus mast cells are activated by IgE-dependent mechanisms to release a variety of preformed and newly generated mediators, which have potent biological effects and are capable of reproducing many of the pathophysiological events seen in acute asthma. The development of antagonists of mast cell derived mediators has so far met with limited success and interpretation of their efficacy is complicated by the multiplicity of mediators released. It is probably too simplistic an approach to expect that antagonism of a single inflammatory mediator will lead to major clinical effects. Nevertheless, some of these newer agents have been shown to attenuate antigen or IgE-dependent bronchial smooth muscle contraction in vitro and asthmatic bronchial reactions in vivo. Although much of this evidence is indirect, taken together it lends considerable weight to the hypothesis that mast cell activation is central in the pathogenesis of asthma.

References

Adams GK, Lichtenstein LM (1979) In vitro studies of antigen-induced bronchospasm: effect of anti- histamines and SRS–A antagonists on the response of sensitised guinea pig and human airways to antigen. J Immunol 122: 555–562
Anwar ARE, Kay AB (1977) The ECF-A tetrapeptides and histamine selectivity enhance human eosinophil complement receptors. Nature 269: 522–524
Atkins PC, Norman M, Weiner H, Zweiman B (1977) Release of neutrophil chemotactic activity during immediate hypersensitivity reactions in humans. Ann Intern Med 86: 415–418
Atkins PC, Norman M, Zweiman B (1978) Antigen-induced chemotactic activity in man: correlation with bronchospasm and inhibition by disodium cromoglycate. J Allergy Clin Immunol 62: 149–155
Austen KF, Brocklehurst WE (1969) Anaphylaxis in chopped guinea pig lung. I. Effect of peptidase substrate and inhibitors. J Exp Med 113: 521–539
Bach MK, Brashler JR, Hammerstrom S, Samuelsson B (1980) Identification of a component of rat mononuclear cell SRS as leukotriene D. Biochem Biophys Res Commun 93: 1121–1126
Boswell RN, Austen KF, Goetzl EJ (1978) Intermediate molecular weight eosinophil chemotactic factors in rat peritoneal mast cells. Immunologic release, granule association and demonstration of structural heterogeneity. J Immunol 120: 15–20
Boucher RC, Ranga V, Pare PD, Inoue S, Moroz L, Hogg JC (1978) Effect of histamine and methacholine on guinea pig tracheal permeability to HRP. J Appl Physiol 45: 939–948
Braude S, Royston D, Coe C, Barnes PJ (1984) Increased lung epithelial permeability to histamine is mediated by H2 receptors. Clin Sci 67: 27p

Brown MJ, Ind PW, Causon R, Lee TH (1982) A novel double isotope technique for the enzymatic assay of plasma histamine: application to estimation of mast cell activation assessed by antigen challenge in asthmatics. J Allergy Clin Immunol 69: 20–24

Bryant DH, Pui A (1982) Histamine content of sputum from patients with asthma and chronic bronchitis. Clin Allergy 12: 19–27

Caulfield JP, Lewis RA, Hein A, Austen KF (1980) Secretion in dissociated human pulmonary mast cells. Evidence for solubilisation of granule contents before discharge. J Cell Biol 85: 299–312

Cazenave JP, Benveniste J, Mustard JF (1979) Aggregation of rabbit platelets by platelet activating factor is independent of the release reaction and the arachidonate pathway and inhibited by membrane active drugs. Lab Invest 41: 275–280

Chakraverty N (1980) The role of plasma membrane calcium-magnesium activated adenosine triphosphate of rat mast cells on histamine release. Acta Pharmacol Toxicol 47: 223–235

Chignard M, Le Coedic JP, Tence M, Vargaftig BB, Benveniste J (1979) The role of platelet activating factor in platelet aggregation. Nature (London) 279: 799–800

Cromwell O, Walport MJ, Taylor GW, Morris HR, O'Driscoll BR, Kay AB (1982) Identification of leukotriene in the sputum of patients with cystic fibrosis. Adv Prostaglandin Thromboxane Leukotriene Res 9: 251

Cutz E, Levison H, Cooper DM (1978) Ultrastructure of airways in children with asthma. Histopathology 2: 407–421

Drazen JM, Schneider MW (1978) Comparative responses of tracheal spirals and parenchymal strips to histamine and carbachol in vivo. J Clin Invest 61: 1441–1447

Dunnill MS (1960) The pathology of asthma with special reference to changes in the bronchial mucosa. J Clin Pathol 13: 27–33

Dunnill MS (1965) Quantitative observations on the anatomy of chronic non-specific lung disease. Med Thorac 22: 261–274

Dunnill MS, Massarella GR, Anderson J (1969) A comparison of quantitative anatomy of the bronchi in normal subjects in status asthmaticus, in chronic bronchitis and emphysema. Thorax 24: 176–179

Earp HS, Steiner AL (1978) Compartmentalisation of cyclic nucleotide-mediated hormone action. Ann Rev Pharmacol Toxicol 18: 431–459

Enerbäck L, Pipkorn U, Granerus U (1986) Intraepithelial migration of nasal mucosal mast cells in hay fever. Int Arch Allergy Appl Immunol 80: 44–51

Goetzl EJ, Austen KF (1975) Purification and synthesis of eosinophilotactic tetrapeptides of human lung tissue: Identification as eosinophilotactic chemotactic factor of anaphylaxis. Proc Natl Acad Sci USA 72: 4123–4127

Green K, Hedquist P, Svanborn N (1974) Increased plasma levels of 15-keto-13, 14-dihydro-prostaglandin F_2 after allergen provoked asthma in man. Lancet II: 1419–1421

Hannsen G, Bjork T, Dahlen SE, Hedqvist P, Granstrom E, Dahlen B (1983) Specific allergen induces contraction of bronchi and formation of leukotriene C4, D4 and E4 in human asthmatic lung. Adv Prostaglandin Thromboxane Leukotriene Res 12: 153–157

Hartley JPR, Nogrady SG (1980) Effects of an inhaled anti-histamine on exercise-induced asthma. Thorax 35: 675–679

Hirata F, Axelrod J (1978) Enzymatic synthesis and rapid translocation of phosphatidyl choline by two methyltransferases in erythrocyte membranes. Proc Natl Acad Sci USA 75: 2348–2352

Hirata F, Axelrod J, Crews FT (1979) Concanavalin A stimulates phospholipid methylation and phosphatidylserine decarboxylation in rat mast cells. Proc Natl Acad Sci USA 76: 4813–4816

Holgate ST, Lewis RA, Austen KF (1980) The role of adenylate cyclase in immunologic release of mediators from rat mast cells: agonist and antagonist effects of purine and ribose modified analogues. Proc Natl Acad Sci USA 77: 6800–6804

Holgate ST, Lewis RA, Maguire JF, Roberts JL II, Oates JA, Austen KF (1980) Effects of prostaglandin D_2 on rat serosal mast cells: Discordance between immunologic mediator release and cyclic AMP levels. J Immunol 125: 1367–1373

Hossain S (1973) Quantitative measurement of bronchial muscle in men with asthma. Am Rev Respir Dis 107: 99–109

Houston JC, de Navasquez S, Trounce JR (1953) A clinical and pathological study of fatal cases of status asthmaticus. Thorax 8: 207–213

Ishizaka T (1981) Analysis of triggering events in mast cells for immunoglobulin E-mediated histamine release. J Allergy Clin Immunol 67: 90–96

Ishizaka T (1982) Biochemical signals induced by bridging of IgE receptors. Fed Proc 14: 17–21

Ishizaka T (1984) IgE-mediated triggering signals for mediator release from human mast cells and basophils. In: Kay AB, Austen KF and Lichtenstein LM (eds). Asthma, physiology, immuno-pharmacology and treatment. Academic Press, London, p 40–51

Ishizaka T, Hirata F, Ishizaka K, Axelrod J (1980) Stimulation of phospholipid methylation, Ca $^{2+}$ influx and histamine release by binding of IgE receptors on rat mast cells. Proc Natl Acad Sci USA 77: 1903–1906

Ishizaka T, Hirata F, Sterk AR, Ishizaka K, Axelrod J (1981) Bridging of IgE receptors activates phospholipid methylation and adenylate cyclase in mast cell plasma membranes. Proc Natl Acad Sci USA 78: 6812–6814

Ishizaka T, Tomioka H, Ishizaka K (1971) Degranulation of human basophil leukocytes by anti-IgE antibody. J Immunol 106: 705–710

Kaliner M, Lemanske R (1984) Mast cell-derived inflammatory factors and late phase allergic reactions. In: Kay AB, Austen KF, Lichtenstein LM (eds) Asthma, physiology, immunopharma-cology and treatment. Academic Press, London, pp 229–242

Kay AB, Austen KF (1971) The IgE-mediated release of an eosinophil leukocyte chemotactic factor from human lung. J Immunol 107: 899–902

Lagunoff D (1974) Histamine binding sites on heparin and mast cell granules. Fed Proc 31: 531 (abstr)

Lee TH, Nagakura T, Cromwell O, Brown MJ, Causon R, Kay AB (1984) Neutrophil chemotactic activity and histamine in atopic and non-atopic subjects after exercise-induced asthma. Am Rev Respir Dis 129: 409–412

Lee TH, Nagy L, Nagakura T, Walport MJ, Kay AB (1982) Identification and partial characterisation of an exercise-induced neutrophil chemotactic factor in bronchial asthma. J Clin Invest 69: 889–99

Levine BB, Fellner MJ (1965) The nature of immune complexes initiating allergic wheal-and-flare reactions. J Allergy 36: 342–352

Lewis RA, Holgate ST, Roberts JL II, Maguire JF, Oates JA, Austen KF (1979) Effects of indomethacin on cyclic nucleotide levels and histamine release from rat serosal mast cells. J Immunol 123: 1663–1668

Lopez-Vidriero MT, Reid L (1983) Pathologic changes in asthma. In: Clark TJH, Godfrey S (eds) Asthma. Chapman and Hall, London, pp 79–99

Loring SH, Drazen JM, Ingram RH (1977) Canine pulmonary response to aerosol histamine: direct verses vagal effect. J Appl Physiol 42: 946–952

Maier M, Spragg J, Schwartz LB (1983) Inactivation of human high molecular weight kininogen by human mast cell tryptase. J Immunol 130: 2352–2356

Marquardt DL, Wasserman SI (1982) Characterisation of the rat mast cell β-adrenergic receptor in resting and stimulated cells by radioligand binding. J Immunol 129: 2122–2126

McLaren K, Holloway, L, Pepper DS (1980) Human platelet factor IV and tissue mast cells. Thrombos Res 19: 293–297

Metcalfe DD, Lewis RA, Silbert JE, Rosenberg RD, Wasserman SI, Austen KF (1979) Isolation and characteristics of heparin from human lung. J Clin Invest 64: 1537–1543

Morris HR, Taylor GW, Clinton PM (1983) Measurement of leukotriene in asthmatics. Adv Prostaglandin, Thromboxane Leukotriene Res ii: 221–223

Morris HR, Taylor GW, Piper PJ, Tippins JR (1980) The structure of slow reacting substance of anaphylaxis from guinea pig lung. Nature (London) 285: 104–105

O'Driscoll BR, Kay AB (1982) Leukotrienes and lung disease. Thorax 37: 241–245

O'Driscoll BR, Lee FH, Cromwell O, Kay AB (1983) Release of high molecular weight neutrophil chemotactic activity (NCA) from immunologically challenged human lung fragments. J Allergy Clin Immunol 71: 146–229

Oertel H, Kaliner M (1981) The biological activity of mast cell granules. II. Purification of inflammatory factors of anaphylaxis (IFA) responsible for causing late phase reactions. J Immunol 127: 1398–1402

Patel KR (1984) Terfenadine in exercise-induced asthma. Br Med J 6429: 1496–1497

Pepys J, Edwards AM (1979) The mast cell, its role in health and disease. Pitman Medical, London

Peters SP, MacGlashan DW, Schulman ES, Schleimer RP, Hayes EC, Rokach J, Adkinson NF, Lichtenstein LM (1984) Arachidonic acid metabolism in purified human lung mast cells. J Immunol 132: 1972–1979

Pietro GC, Magno M (1978) Pharmacologic factors influencing permeability of the bronchial microcirculation. Fed Proc 37: 2466–2470

Plaut M, Lichtenstein LM, Gillespie E, Henney CS (1973) Studies on the mechanisms of lymphocyte mediated cytolysis IV: Specificity of the histamine receptor on effector T cells. J Immunol III: 389– 394

Rocklin RE, Haberek-Davidson E (1981) Histamine activates suppressor cells in vitro using a coculture technique. J Clin Immunol 1: 73–79

Salvato G (1968) Some histological changes in chronic bronchitis and asthma. Thorax 23: 168–172

Schechter NM, Fraki JE, Geesin JC, Lazarus GS (1983) Human skin chymotryptic protease. Isolation and relation to cathepsin g and rat mast cell proteinase I. J Biol Chem 258: 2973–2978

Schild HO, Hawkins DF, Mongar JL, Herxheimer H (1951) Reactions of isolated human asthmatic lung and bronchus tissue to a specific antigen. Lancet II: 376–382

Schwartz LB, Austen KF, Wasserman SI (1979) Immunologic release of hexosaminadase and glucuronidase from purified rat serosal mast cells. J Immunol 123: 1445–1450

Schwartz LB, Kawahari MS, Hugh TE, Vik D, Fearon DT, Austen KF (1983) Generation of C3a anaphylotoxin from human C3 by human mast cell tryptase. J Immunol 130: 1891–1895

Schwartz LB, Lewis RA, Seldin D, Austen KF (1981) Acid hydrolases and tryptase from secretory granules of dispersed human lung mast cells. J Immunol 126: 1290–1294

Shelhamer JH, Marom Z, Kaliner M (1980) Immunologic and neuropharmacologic stimulation of mucous glycoprotein release from human airways in vitro. J Clin Invest 66: 1400–1408

Tannenbaum S, Oertel H, Henderson W, Kaliner M (1980) The biological activity of mast cell granules. I. Elicitation of inflammatory responses in rat skin. J Immunol 125: 325–335

Tigelaar RE, Vaz NM, Ovary Z (1971) Immunoglobulin receptors on mouse mast cells. J Immunol 106: 661–672

Turnbull LS, Turnbull LW, Leitch AG, Crofton JW, Kay AB (1977) Mediators of immediate hypersensitivity in sputum of patients with chronic bronchitis and asthma. Lancet II: 526–529

Turner-Warwick M (1978) Immunology of the lung. Edward Arnold, London.

Uvnas B, Aborg CH (1977) On the cation exchange properties of rat mast cell granules and their storage of histamine. Acta Physiol Scand 100: 309–314

Uvnas B, Aborg CH, Begendorff A (1970) Storage of histamine in mast cells. Evidence for an ionic binding of histamine to protein carboxyls in the granule heparin-protein complex. Acta Physiol Scand 78 (Suppl) 336: 1–26

Warner JO (1978) Significance of late reactions after bronchial challenge with house dust mite. Arch Dis Child 51: 905–911

Winslow CM, Austen KF (1982) Enzymatic regulation of mast cell activation and secretion by adenylate cyclase and cyclic AMP-dependent protein kinases. Fed Proc 41: 22–29

Woenne R, Katten M, Orange RP, Levison H (1978) Bronchial hyperreactivity to histamine and methacholine in asthmatic children after inhalation of Sch 1000 and chlorpheniramine maleate. J Allergy Clin Immunol 62: 119–124

Chapter 2

Mast Cell Heterogeneity

Mast cells were first described by Erhlich in 1877, at which time he named them *"Mastzellen"* or well-fed cells because of the prominent granules in their cytoplasm. They may be recognised by these large electron dense cytoplasmic granules which stain metachromatically with conventional cationic dyes such as toluidine blue (Seyle 1965). However, it is important to recognise that mast cells from different species and even from different tissues within the same species exhibit marked variations in their morphological and functional properties (Pearce et al. 1982b).

Morphological Heterogeneity

Maximov as long ago as 1904 designated certain mast cells in the rat intestinal mucosa as atypical. This work was extended by Enerback (1966a, b) in an elegant study demonstrating that the properties of staining and fixation of mast cells in the gastrointestinal mucosa (mucosal or atypical mast cells) differed from those widely distributed in connective tissues (connective tissue mast cells). He showed that the mucosal mast cell of the rat small intestine was well preserved after fixation in Carnoy's fluid (ethanol : chloroform : acetic acid, 6:3:1) but that the cytoplasmic granules failed to stain after fixation in conventional aldehyde fixatives. The structure of the connective tissue mast cell was well preserved by both methods of fixation (Enerback 1966a). When sections were stained with alcian blue and then counterstained with safranin in the alcian blue–safranin reaction, mast cells in the rat gastrointestinal mucosa retained the alcian blue in their granules. These mucosal mast cells were therefore alcian blue positive. However, the alcian blue was displaced from the granules of the connective tissue mast cell by the safranin. Thus, connective tissue mast cells were safranin positive. In addition, the rat connective tissue mast cell granule takes up the fluorescent cationic dye, berberine sulphate, resulting in a bright yellow fluorescence. This dye, which preferentially binds to heparin, is not taken up by the granules of mucosal mast cells (Enerback and Wingren 1980). A similar differential effect of fixation has been demonstrated in mast cells in the human jejunal mucosa (Strobel et al. 1981).

Table 2.1. Morphological heterogeneity of mast cells

	Mucosal mast cell	Connective tissue mast cell
Fixation		
Carnoy's	+	+
Formol saline	−	+
Staining		
Alcian blue	+	−
Safranin 0	−	+
Berberine sulphate	−	+
Immunohistochemical		
Intracellular IgE	+	−
RMCP	II	I

The observed differences in the conditions of staining and fixation (Table 2.1) between connective tissue and mucosal mast cells have been attributed to the presence of different glycosaminoglycans in the two cell types (Enerback 1966a, b; Tas 1977; Tas and Bernsden 1977). Combs et al. (1965) observed a shift from preferential staining with alcian blue to preferential staining with safranin 0 in mast cell granules of rat embryos, dependent upon their maturity. Cells with alcian blue positive granules were present in early gestation but were almost entirely replaced by safranin positive cells at full term. This shift in staining characteristics occurred in parallel with the increasing sulphation of the glycosaminoglycan as the cells matured, suggesting that alcian blue stained immature precursor cells containing poorly sulphated glycosaminoglycans. However, the fixative used (neutral buffered formalin) was unlikely to preserve the mucosal mast cell population and no similar shift from alcian blue to safranin positivity has been observed during the differentiation of rat intestinal mucosal mast cells from lymphoblast-like precursors during parasitic infestation (Miller 1971). That the rat mucosal mast cell does not contain heparin but contains a glycosaminoglycan of a lower degree of sulphation has been confirmed by microspectroscopic analysis (Tas and Bernsden 1977). However, it is unlikely that the differences in fixation and staining are wholly attributable to the degree of sulphation of the glycosaminoglycan. Mucosal mast cells can be stained in aldehyde-fixed tissues after very long staining times and partial restoration of staining even with short staining times can be achieved by treatment of sections with trypsin (Wingren and Enerback 1983). This is more consistent with the hypothesis that these differences are due to differences in the glycosaminogly-can–protein complexes. Aldehydes combine with cationic protein groups forming crosslinks between polypeptide chains (Pearse 1968). Aldehyde fixation may therefore create a protein shell shielding the glycosaminoglycan and its dye-binding sulphate groups.

There is also evidence that rat mast cells contain different proteases dependent upon their location. Rat mast cell protease I has been identified immunohistochemically in mast cells from the peritoneal cavity (Yurt and Austen 1977), skin (Seppa and Jarvinen 1978) and muscle (Woodbury et al. 1978a). Mucosal mast cells of the gastrointestinal tract contain an immunologi-cally distinct protease termed rat mast cell protease II (Woodbury et al. 1978b). Both have chymotryptic activity.

An additional difference concerns the histamine content of these two mast cell subpopulations. Parallel mast cell counts and histamine assays in different tissues indicate that the histamine content of the mucosal mast cell is considerably lower than that of the connective tissue mast cell—about 1 pg/cell compared with 10 pg/cell (Enerback and Wingren 1980). Finally, there is some evidence that mucosal mast cells of the rat intestine contain intracellular IgE, unlike connective tissue mast cells where IgE is confined to cell surface receptors (Mayrhofer et al. 1976).

Ontogeny of Mast Cells

The ontogeny of mucosal and connective tissue mast cells may be distinct (Fig. 2.1). The mucosal mast cell hyperplasia which occurs during infestation with nematodes such as the intestinal parasite *Nippostrongylus brasiliensis* is dependent upon the integrity of the host T-cell system. It does not occur in T-cell depleted rodents (Mayrhofer and Fisher 1979) nor in nude mice (Ruitenberg and Elgersma 1976). The observation that during this hyperplasia, mucosal mast cells differentiate from cells indistinguishable from lymphoblasts (Miller 1971) suggested that they may be T-cell derived. However, it is possible to transfer the mastopoietic response with immune serum which would suggest that masto-poiesis is dependent upon T-cell factor (Befus and Bienenstock 1979). This hypothesis is supported by the culture of mast cells in vitro from rodent bone marrow. Mast cells multiply to predominance in long term bone marrow cultures under the influence of a T-cell derived lymphokine (Haig et al. 1982) putatively interleukin 3 (Ihle et al. 1983). Such cultured mast cells have similar properties of staining and fixation to rodent intestinal mucosal mast cells (Haig et al. 1982; Sredni et al. 1983) and contain chondroitin sulphate E rather than heparin proteoglycan (Razin et al. 1982b).

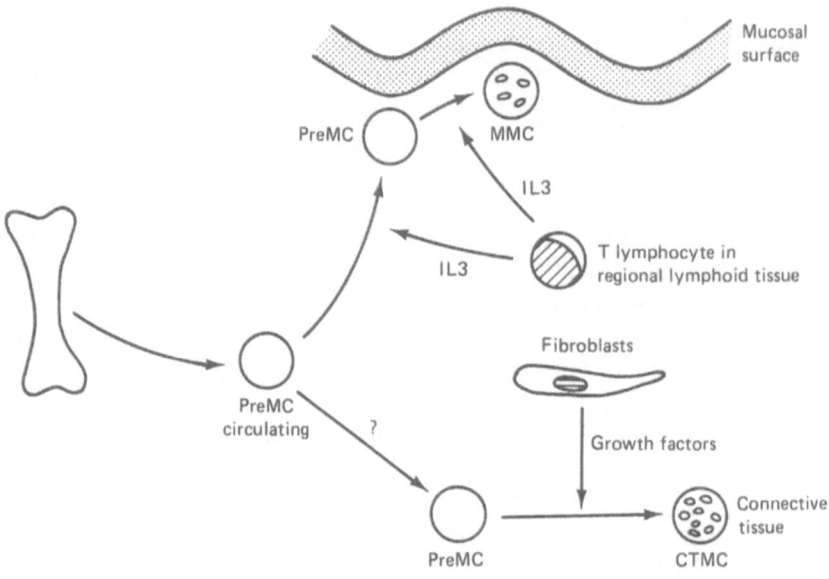

Fig. 2.1. Mast cell development. *PreMC*, mast cell precursor; *MMC*, mucosal mast cell; *CTMC*, connective tissue mast cell; *IL3*, interleukin 3.

Connective tissue mast cells were originally thought to differentiate in situ from connective tissue elements but it now seems likely that these too are derived from bone marrow (Kitimura et al. 1979). The connective tissue mast cell system does not appear to be T-cell dependent and the factor or factors controlling the differentiation and distribution of connective tissue mast cells remain unidentified. More recently, work from the same laboratory has provided evidence for a common precursor for both mast cell types. Mast cells derived in vitro from rodent bone marrow were injected intravenously, intraperitoneally or intradermally into mast cell deficient mice. These cells were capable of repopulating both connective tissue and mucosal sites with the classical mucosal or connective tissue type of mast cell. Surprisingly, they also showed that peritoneal cells from syngeneic mice were also capable of repopulating mucosal sites in mast cell deficient mice suggesting the presence of precursors in the peritoneal cavity capable of differentiating into mucosal mast cells (Nakano et al. 1985).

Repeated injections of the polyamine 48/80 leads to discharge of connective tissue mast cell granules and the proliferation of mucosal mast cells of the rat intestinal tract. Using the rate of disappearance of these newly formed mucosal mast cells Enerback and Lowhagen (1979) calculated that the life span of the mucosal mast cell is approximately 40 days. In contrast, connective tissue mast cells are long lived, with little turnover in terms of cell death and renewal (Padawer 1974). It remains possible therefore that differences between mucosal and connective tissue mast cells are related to the relative immaturity of the former population.

Two other morphologically distinct cells with metachromatic granules have been identified in the rat gastrointestinal mucosa. The globule leucocyte contains many granules with high affinity for the cationic dyes and lies superficially within the mucosa, above the basement membrane and between the epithelial cells (Huntley et al. 1984). The granular intraepithelial lymphocytes appear as lymphocytes within the epithelium but contain a few polar metachromatic granules. In the rat, all three—mucosal mast cells, globule leucocytes and granular intraepithelial lymphocytes—contain glycosaminoglycan and serine esterase. Mucosal mast cells and globule leucocytes contain rat mast cell protease II and the globule leucocyte probably represents a mucosal mast cell which has migrated into the epithelium (Huntley et al. 1984). The relationship of granular intraepithelial lymphocytes to the mast cell system is uncertain (Ferguson 1977).

Functional Differences

Given the widespread distribution of mast cells, it is fundamental to our understanding of the aetiology and prophylaxis of allergic conditions to appreciate that mastocytes from different locations may show marked variations in their functional characteristics. Large numbers of mast cells which occur in the serosal cavities of rodents, particularly the rat, may be isolated by simple lavage. As a result, much of our knowledge of mast cell function is based upon studies of the rat peritoneal mast cell (Table 2.2).

The classical mast cell secretagogue, compound 48/80, causes a rapid release of histamine from rat peritoneal mast cells. Enerback (1966c) made the original

Table 2.2. Functional heterogeneity of mast cells

	Mucosal mast cell	Connective tissue mast cell
Histamine	+	++
Secretagogues		
48/80	−	+
Peptide 401	−	+
Anti-allergics		
DSCG	−	+
Theophylline	−	+
Newly generated mediators		
PGD_2	+[a]	+++
LTC_4	+++[a]	+

[a]Data refer to mast cells cultured in vitro from rodent bone marrow under the influence of T cell factors.

observation that mucosal mast cells of the rat gastrointestinal tract were unaffected by this polyamine. Since then, techniques have been developed to disperse cells from intact tissues by a combination of mechanical disruption and enzymic digestion (Paterson et al. 1976). The preparations of mast cells thus obtained appear to be morphologically intact and biochemically unimpaired (Peters et al. 1982). It has now been possible, therefore, to confirm using in vitro cell suspensions this lack of responsiveness of the rat gastrointestinal mucosal mast cell to the classic secretagogues polyamine 48/80 and bee venom peptide 401 (Befus et al. 1982). The mucosal mast cell in this species is, in addition, refractory to the inhibitory effects of sodium cromoglycate and theophylline, unlike the peritoneal mast cell (Pearce et al. 1982). In the last few years the response of mast cells obtained from different species to a wide variety of histamine liberators and anti-anaphylactic compounds has been investigated. A spectrum of response is apparent (Ennis and Pearce 1980). A similar spectrum of response has been demonstrated using mast cells dispersed from different sites in a single species (Pearce et al. 1982b).

Further evidence of functional mast cell heterogeneity has been derived from comparisons between rat serosal heparin containing mast cells and mouse bone marrow derived mast cells which contain chondroitin-sulphate E proteoglycan.

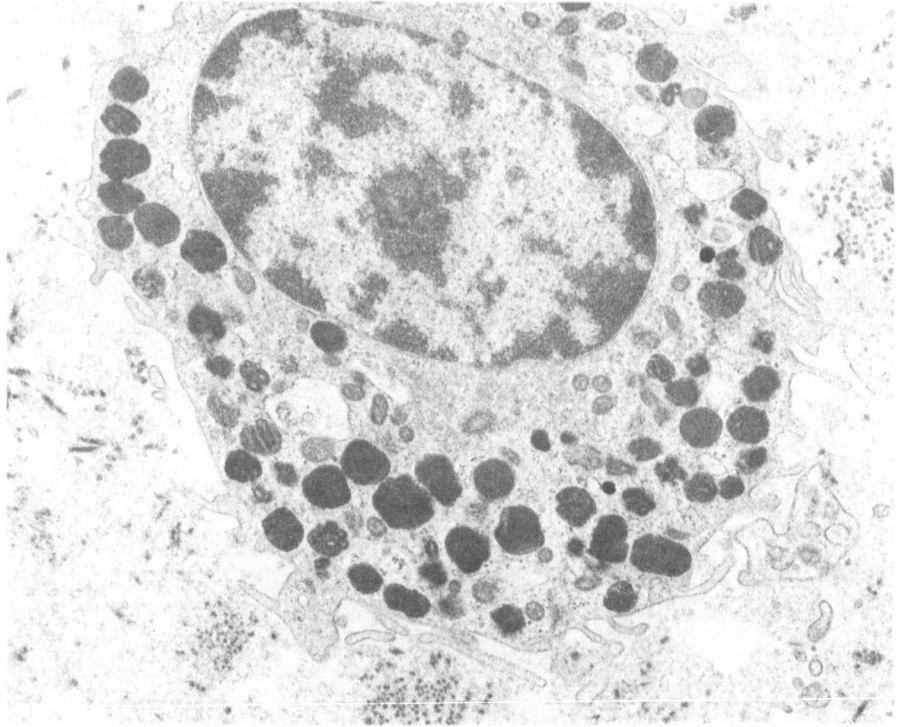

Fig. 2.2. Electron micrograph of a mast cell isolated from lamina propria of human bronchus.

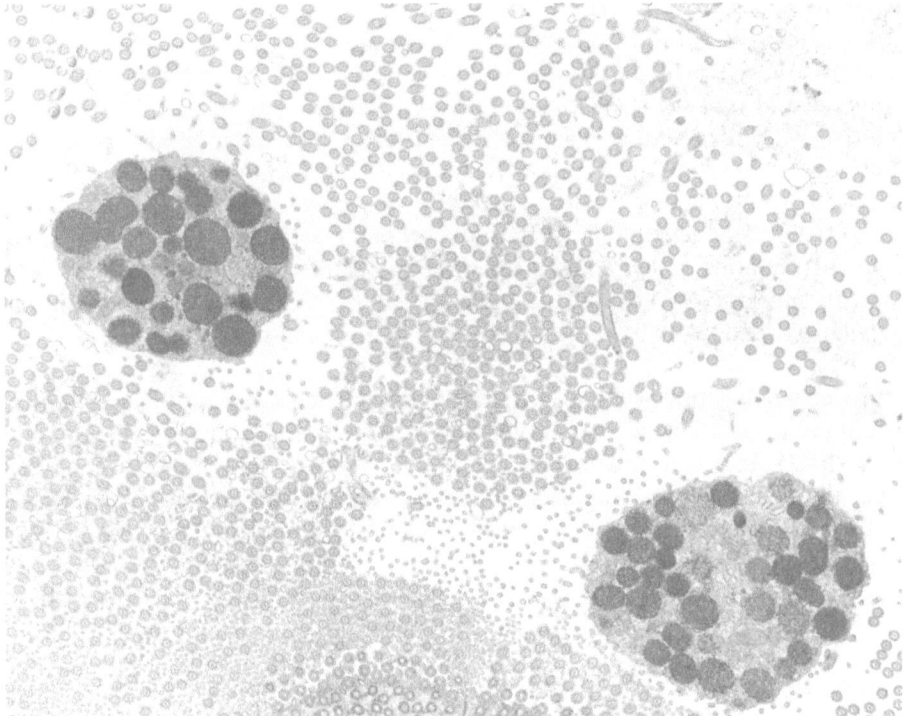

Fig. 2.3. Electron micrograph showing two mast cells lying superficially among the cilia of human bronchial epithelium.

Both, like all other mast cells so far identified, will release histamine after IgE-dependent immunological challenge. However, after activation, the rat serosal mast cell generates prostaglandin D_2 (PGD_2) as its major cyclooxygenase product with little generation of leukotriene C4 (Lewis et al. 1982). Conversely, the in vitro bone marrow derived mast cell generates substantial amounts of leukotriene C_4 (LTC_4) and little PGD_2 (Razin et al. 1982a). Thus, although the in vivo counterpart of this bone marrow derived mast cell has not been conclusively determined, it seems that the spectrum of mediators released after activation of different mast cell subtypes is likely to be different.

Human lung mast cells may similarly be obtained in single cell suspensions using a combination of mechanical disruption and enzymic digestion (Paterson et al. 1976). Heterogeneity of this mast cell population has been demonstrated both ultrastructurally, and on the basis of size and histamine release. The major type of dispersed lung mast cell has granules with crystalline contents (scrolls, gratings or lattices) which become amorphous on activation (Fig. 2.2) whilst other cells contain predominantly granules which have an amorphous structure in the absence of stimulation (Fig. 2.3) (Caulfield et al. 1980; Brinkman 1968). Partial purification of human lung mast cells after dispersion may be achieved by countercurrent centrifugal elutriation (Schulman et al. 1982). This technique separates cells according to size and density, yielding mast cells of differing size and histamine content in different fractions and varying from 2 pg/cell in the smallest to 15 pg/cell in the largest (Schulman et al. 1983). This difference between the large and small cells extends to mediator release. The smaller cells respond poorly to IgE-mediated signals, releasing a lower percentage of histamine (and therefore a lower absolute amount) and less PGD_2 (Schulman et al. 1983).

There are conflicting reports concerning the generation of sulphidopeptide leukotriene by partially purified human lung mast cells. Cells purified by gradient methods yield reduced quantities of leukotriene, measured as slow reacting substance of anaphylaxis (SRSA) relative to histamine than the initial population leading to speculation that a second non-mast cell type may be involved (Lewis et al. 1981). However when purified by countercurrent centrifugal elutriation, yielding fractions of varying mast cell purity and number, histamine release purifies in parallel with leukotriene generation (MacGlashan et al. 1982). It is conceivable that rather than a requirement for a second cell type, the two methods are purifying different subpopulations of mast cells and that there exists in human lung a mast cell subclass comparable to that derived from rodent bone marrow.

References

Befus AD, Bienenstock J (1979) Immunologically-mediated intestinal mastocytes in *Nippostrongylus brasiliensis*-infected rats. Immunology 38: 95–101

Befus AD, Pearce FL, Gauldie J, Horsewood P, Bienenstock J (1982) I. Isolation and functional characteristics of rat intestinal mast cells. J Immunol 128: 2475–2480

Brinkman L (1968) The mast cell in normal human bronchus and lung. J Ultrastruct Res 23: 115–123

Caulfield JP, Lewis RA, Hein A, Austen KF (1980) Secretion in dissociated human pulmonary mast cells. Evidence for solubilisation of granule contents before discharge. J Cell Biol 85: 299–312

Combs JW, Lagunoff D, Benditt EP (1965) Differentiation and proliferation of the embryonic mast cells of the rat. J Cell Biol 25: 577–592

Enerback L (1966a) Mast cells in the rat gastrointestinal mucosa. I. Effects of fixation. Acta Pathol Microbiol Scand 66: 289–302

Enerback L (1966b) Mast cells in the rat gastrointestinal mucosa. II. Dye-binding and metachromatic properties. Acta Pathol Microbiol Scand 66:303–312

Enerback L (1966c) Mast cells in rat gastrointestinal mucosa. III. Reactivity towards compound 48/80. Acta Pathol Microbiol Scand 66: 312–322

Enerback L, Lowhagen GB (1979) Long term increase of mucosal mast cells in the rat induced by administration of compound 48/80. Cell Tissue Res 198: 209–215

Enerback L, Wingren U (1980) Histamine content of peritoneal and tissue mast cells of growing rats. Histochemistry 66: 113–124

Ennis M, Pearce FL (1980) Differential reactivity of isolated mast cells from the rat and guinea pig. Eur J Pharmacol 66: 339–345

Erhlich P (1877) Arch Micros Anat 13: 263–277. Quoted in Heatley RV (1983) The gastrointestinal mucosal mast cell. Scand J Gastroenterol 185: 449–453

Ferguson A (1977) Intraepithelial lymphocytes of the small intestine. Gut 18: 921–937

Haig DM, McKee TA, Jarrett EEE, Woodbury R, Miller HRP (1982) Generation of mucosal mast cells is stimulated in vitro by factors derived from T-cells of helminth infected rats. Nature 300: 188–190

Huntley JF, McGorum B, Newlands GFJ, Miller HRP (1984) Granular intraepithelial lymphocytes: their relationship to mucosal mast cells and globule leucocytes. Immunology 53: 525–535

Ihle JN, Keller J, Oroszlan S et al. (1983) Biologic properties of homogeneous interleukin 3. I. Demonstration of WeHI 3 growth factor activity, mast cell growth factor activity, P cell stimulating factor activity and histamine producing cell stimulating factor activity. J Immunol 131: 382–387

Kitimura Y, Matsuda H, Hatanaka K (1979) Clonal nature of mast cell clusters formed in W/WV mice after bone marrow transplantation. Nature 281: 154–155

Lewis RA, Drazen JM, Corey EJ, Austen KF (1981) Structural and functional characteristics of the leukotriene components of slow reacting substance of anaphylaxis (SRS-A) In: PJ Piper (ed) SRS-A and the leukotrienes. Wiley, London pp 101–117

Lewis RA, Soter NA, Diamond PT, Austen KF, Oates JA, Roberts LJ (1982) Prostaglandin D_2 generation after activation of rat and human mast cells with anti-IgE. J Immunol 129: 1627–1631

MacGlashan DW, Schleimer RP, Peters SP et al. (1982) Generation of leukotrienes by purified human lung mast cells. J Clin Invest 70: 747–751

Maximov A (1904) Uber die Zellformen deslockeren bindergewebes. Arch fuer Mikrosk Anat und Entwicklungsmechanik 67: 680–757

Mayrhofer G, Fisher R (1979) Mast cells in severely T-cell depleted rats and response to infestation with *Nippostrongylus brasiliensis*. Immunology 37: 145–155

Mayrhofer G, Bazin H, Cowans JL (1976) The nature of cells binding IgE in rats immunised with *Nippostrongylus brasiliensis*. I. IgE synthesis in regional nodes and concentration in mucosal mast cells. Eur J Immunol 6: 537–545

Miller HRP (1971) Immune reactions in mucous membranes. II. The differentiation of intestinal mast cells during helminth expulsion in the rat. Lab Invest 24: 339–347

Nakano T, Sonoda T, Hayashi C et al. (1985) Fate of bone marrow-derived cultured mast cells after intracutaneous, intraperitoneal and intravenous transfer into genetically mast cell deficient W/Wv mice. J Exp Med 162: 1025–1043

Padawer J (1974) Mast cells. Extended life span and lack of granule turnover under normal in vivo conditions. Exp Molec Path 20: 269–280

Paterson NAM, Wasserman SI, Said JW, Austen KF (1976) Release of chemical mediators from partially purified human lung mast cells. J Immunol 117: 1356–1362

Pearce FL, Befus AD, Bienenstock J (1982a) Isolation and properties of mast cells from the small bowel lamina propria of the rat. Agents and Actions 12: 183–185

Pearce FL, Befus AD, Gauldie J, Bienenstock J (1982b) Mucosal mast cells. II. Effects of anti-allergic compounds on histamine secretion by isolated intestinal mast cells. J Immunol 128: 2481–2486

Pearse AGE (1968) Histochemistry, theoretical and applied, 3rd edn. Churchill Livingstone, London, pp 70–76

Peters SP, Schulman ES, Schleimer RP, MacGlashan DW, Newball HH, Lichtenstein LM (1982) Dispersed human lung mast cells. Pharmacologic aspects and comparison with human lung tissue fragments. Am Rev Resp Dis 126: 1034–1039

Peters SP, MacGlashan DW, Schulman ES, Schleimer RP, Hayes EC, Rokach J, Adkinson NF, Lichtenstein LM (1984) Arachidonic acid metabolism in purified human lung mast cells. J Immunol 132: 1972–1979

Razin E, Mencia-Huerta JM, Lewis RA, Corey EJ, Austen KF (1982a) Generation of leukotriene C4 from a subclass of mast cells differentiated in vitro from mouse bone marrow. Proc Natl Acad Sci USA 79: 4665–4667

Razin E, Stevens RL, Akiyama F, Schmid L, Austen KF (1982b) Culture from mouse bone marrow of a subclass of mast cells possessing a distinct chondroitin sulphate proteoglycan with glycosaminoglycans rich in N-acetyl-galactosamine-4,6-disulphate. J Biol Chem 257: 7229–7236

Razin E, Mencia-Huerta JM, Stevens RL, Lewis RA, Lui FT, Corey EJ, Austen KF (1983) IgE mediated release of leukotriene C4, chondroitin sulphate E proteoglycan, β-hexosaminadase and histamine from cultured bone marrow derived mouse mast cells. J Exp Med 157: 189–201

Ruitenberg EJ, Elgersma A (1976) Absence of intestinal mast cell response in congenitally athymic mice during *Trichinella spiralis* infection. Nature 264: 256–260

Schulman ES, MacGlashan DW, Peters SP, Schleimer RP, Newball H, Lichtenstein LM (1982) Human lung mast cells: purification and characterisation. J Immunol 129: 2662–2667

Schulman ES, Kagey-Sabotka A, MacGlashan DW et al. (1983) Heterogeneity of human lung mast cells. J Immunol 131: 1936–1941

Seppa HEJ, Jarvinen M (1978) Rat skin main neutral protease: purification and properties. J Invest Dermatol 70: 84–89

Seyle H (1965) The mast cells. Butterworth, Washington

Sredni B, Freedman MM, Bland CE, Metcalfe DD (1983) Ultrastructural, biochemical and functional characteristics of histamine-containing cells cloned from mouse bone marrow: tentative identification as mucosal mast cells. J Immunol 131: 915–922

Strobel S, Miller HRP, Ferguson A (1981) Human intestinal mucosal mast cells: evaluation of fixation and staining techniques. J Clin Pathol 34: 851–858

Tas J (1977) The alcian blue and combined alcian blue—safranin staining of glycosaminoglycans studied in a model system and in mast cells. Histochem J 9: 205–230

Tas J, Bernsden RG (1977) Does heparin occur in mucosal mast cells of the rat small intestine? J Histochem Cytochem 25: 1058–1062

Wingren W, Enerback L (1983) Mucosal mast cells of the rat intestine: a re-evaluation of fixation and staining properties with special reference to protein blocking and solubility of the glycosaminoglycan. Histochem J 15: 571–582

Woodbury RG, Everitt M, Sandada Y, Katunuma N, Lagunoff D, Neuraff H (1978a) Major serine protease in rat skeletal muscle: evidence for its mast cell origin. Proc Natl Acad Sci USA 75: 5311–5313

Woodbury RG, Gruzenski DM, Lagunoff D (1978b) Immunofluorescent localisation of a serine protease in rat small intestine. Proc Natl Acad Sci USA 75: 2785–2789

Yurt R, Austen KF (1977) Preparative purification of the rat mast cell chymase. Characterisation and interaction with granule components. J Exp Med 146: 1405–1419

Chapter 3

Superficial Mast Cells and the Asthmatic Response

Introduction

There are few quantitative studies of the distribution of mast cells in human lung. Brinkman (1968) found mast cells within the bronchial mucosa but felt that these were rare in comparison with submucosal mast cells. In a systematic study of mast cells in the lungs of the monkey, *Macaca fasicularis*, Guerzon et al. (1979) confirmed that the majority of lung mast cells did indeed lie in the submucosa. However, they found significant numbers of mast cells lying within the mucosa between the epithelial cells; they calculated that 83% of mast cells were associated with conducting airways and an average of 12% of these were mucosal. Perhaps more significantly, not only did the total number of mast cells in the mucosa and the submucosa increase greatly towards the periphery but also the proportion of mucosal to submucosal cells increased from only 0.4% in the trachea to up to 27% in bronchioles.

In asthmatic lungs, Cutz et al. (1978) have identified intramucosal mast cells by electron microscopy. In lung biopsies from two asthmatic subjects in remission and two who died in status asthmaticus, the intramucosal mast cells appeared in varying stages of degranulation whereas the submucosal mast cells remained packed with homogeneous electron dense granules. The pattern of degranulation suggests a differential stability of the mucosal and submucosal cells. Salvato (1968) attempted a comparison of mast cell numbers in the lungs of control subjects and those with bronchial asthma. He showed a reduction in the number of mast cells in the asthmatic lung with marked degranulation of the remaining mast cells. This he felt was consistent with a failure to identify completely degranulated mast cells using conventional light microscopy.

Sir John Floyer (1698) in one of the earliest descriptions of asthma was well aware of the speed with which an asthmatic attack may develop. With the advent of bronchial provocation testing this observation has been confirmed many times in the standardised conditions of the laboratory. Inhaled antigens are known to be large molecular weight particles (Findlay et al. 1983) and the majority of mast cells identified within human lung lie in the airway submucosa (Guerzon et al. 1979; Brinkman 1968). It seems unlikely therefore that inhaled antigen can penetrate into small airways and cross the airway mucosa to reach these submucosal mast cells in the short space of time taken to generate a bronchoconstrictor response. This is particularly true considering the demonstrated impermeability of the bronchial mucosa to large molecular weight substances (Simani et al. 1974). Consideration of these facts led Hogg and co-workers to propose that the rapid response occurring in allergic individuals might be due to an interaction between antigen and mast cells lying superficially in the bronchial mucosa or free within the airway lumen (Hogg et al. 1977).

Thus the initial interaction between antigen and mast cell bound IgE may occur at or near the airway surface. In view of the considerable evidence of mast cell heterogeneity, this population of mast cells, lying superficially within the bronchial mucosa or free within the bronchial lumen, may possess properties which are quite distinct from the majority found within the human lung.

Bronchoalveolar Lavage Technique

The technique of bronchoalveolar lavage is now a well established method of recovery of both cells and fluid for clinical and research purposes. However, as the results of this work are now being published, many apparent discrepancies between different groups are seen (Flint et al. 1985a). One possible reason for these discrepancies could be small variations of bronchoalveolar lavage technique used by the different groups engaged in this work. It is also important to remember that the technique of bronchoalveolar lavage carries with it a certain risk especially when asthmatic patients are involved, and so patient selection should be done with great care.

In general most groups involved in this work use similar methods, that is, sterile physiological saline is introduced into a lobe of the lung through the biopsy channel of a fibreoptic bronchoscope which has been gently wedged into a midsize bronchus. The saline wash is then recovered by gentle suction. The saline can be shown to reach the alveoli distal to the bronchoscope but it is not known if the recovered sample would include material found at such a distance from the tip of the bronchoscope.

The volume of saline used per site has been shown to be important. Most reported studies have used between 100 ml and 150 ml, which is infused in aliquots of 20–50 ml. It is generally agreed that the first of these aliquots washes out a different population of cells than the subsequent washes. The first wash contains cells recovered proximally to the bronchoscope and the further washes reach more distal regions. This difference in differential cell recovery was confirmed in a study I carried out using a bronchoscope fitted with a balloon which enabled me to make a distal and a proximal lavage. In general I recovered more epithelial and dead cells from the proximal airways lavage. These findings lead some groups to discard the first aliquot whilst other groups argue that this first sample accounts for such a small percent of the whole lavage it will make little or no difference to the lavage overall; in my work I have used the whole lavage. Most of the groups, including myself, have found that two separate lobes can be lavaged using a total volume of up to 320 ml and this, in my experience, causes no clinical problems. Using volumes in excess of 320 ml or more than two lobes in most cases leads to a transient fever. In my experience, no other significant complication is involved with the technique.

The lavage fluid should be collected into siliconised glass bottles and processed as soon as possible. The collection bottle is usually kept on ice but we found that although this had little or no effect on the cell number or differential of the recovered sample, it could adversely effect the function of the cells. I found that the mast cells recovered from asthmatic subjects spontaneously released histamine to a greater level than the controls, and if the cells were kept at 4°C this could represent almost 100% release of this mediator, thus making it impossible to do functional studies. Therefore we collected our samples at room temperature.

Most groups wash the cells and then make cytocentrifuge preparations which are then fixed and stained for differential counting using Wright-Giemsa or a similar stain, but a number of groups have shown this can distort the actual differential and total cell recovery and they favour other methods of lavage processing, for example filtration on to millipore filters. However, it is generally agreed that for most purposes the cytocentrifuge method is adequate (Crystal et al. 1986).

Bronchoalveolar lavage (BAL) is now accepted as a useful and safe technique with most patient groups tolerating the procedure well. However, there are certain contraindications: for example, an $FEV_1<1$ litre, a $PaO_2<60$ mmHg, myocardial infarction, angina, congestive cardiac failure and severe intercurrent illness.

The method of BAL I adopted was performed using a technique modified from the original description of Reynolds and Newball (1974). Patients were premedicated using intravenous atropine (0.6 mg), diazemuls (5–15 mg) or midazolam (2.5–10 mg) and fentanyl (100 mg). Local anaesthesia of the nose and pharynx was obtained using 10% lignocaine spray. The fibreoptic bronchoscope (an Olympus BF2 ITR or IT10) was then passed via the nose and 2 ml of 4% lignocaine instilled over the vocal cords. Three further aliquots of 2% lignocaine were instilled, one into the trachea, one into the right and one into the left main bronchi. The tip of the fibreoptic bronchoscope was then wedged into the subsegmental bronchus to be lavaged, usually the medial segment of the right middle lobe or lingula or the medial segment of the right or left lower lobe.

Three 60 ml aliquots of normal saline (0.9% w/v), buffered to pH 7.4 by the addition of 0.275 ml sodium bicarbonate 8.4%/500 ml and prewarmed to 37°C, were then instilled sequentially into the lung subsegment. The bronchoscope was then disimpacted and the fluid recovered by gentle aspiration (ca. 100 mmHg) into siliconised glass containers. The recovered lavage fluid was centrifuged and the fluid decanted from the cells. The cells were washed twice with RPMI-1640 culture medium and resuspended in 5 ml of medium for total and viable cell counts. This procedure was modified slightly in asthmatic subjects. Once below the vocal cords, only isotonic prewarmed lignocaine solution (xylocaine epidural 1.5%) was used, and supplementary oxygen was given via a nasal catheter during the lavage procedure. After the lavage, the asthmatics received nebulised salbutamol and hydrocortisone (100 mg/iv). Fluid recovery from lower lobes in asthmatic subjects was poor and therefore in these subjects BAL was confined to the right middle lobe. In control subjects for these studies bronchoalveolar cells were handled in exactly the same way.

Human Bronchoalveolar and Dispersed Lung Mast Cells

Until recently the only available in vitro model of human mast cell function was the human dispersed cell preparation. Free cells can be obtained from human lung fragments by a combination of mechanical disruption and enzymic digestion (Paterson et al. 1976). Dispersed cell preparations contain between 1% and 8% mast cells which appear to be functionally intact in that their responses resemble those of the intact tissues (Peters et al. 1982). Such cells are dispersed from throughout the lung parenchyma, and as the majority of mast cells lie in perivascular and submucosal connective tissues, it is presumably these that make the major contribution to this preparation. These dispersed human lung mast cell preparations have been widely used as an in vitro model of asthma, but the properties of mast cells dispersed from tissues deep within the lung may not be relevant to the initial events which follow the inhalation of antigen.

Mast cells lying superficially have been obtained from primate lungs by bronchoalveolar lavage. In rhesus monkeys, Patterson and co-workers in the mid-1970s recovered cells resembling mast cells and basophils by saline lobar lavage (Patterson et al. 1974). These cells were capable of histamine release in response to anti-IgE or specific ascaris antigen; transfer of cells recovered from the bronchial lumen of an ascaris antigen sensitive donor monkey to a non-sensitive recipient, transferred an antigen specific bronchial reaction (Patterson et al. 1978). Similar cells were demonstrated in human lungs by limited lavage of central airways but functional studies were complicated by high rates of spontaneous histamine release (Patterson et al. 1977).

The introduction of fibre-optic bronchoscopy and the subsequent development of BAL has provided a new approach to the investigation of many respiratory disorders. It allows the recovery of living human lung cells for study in vitro providing a window through which we can examine human mucosal defence mechanisms. The recovered lavage fluid contains soluble proteins and electrolytes of the lung secretions and cells from the lung surface. The cell types recovered vary, depending upon the type of subjects lavaged. Total and differential cell counts in BAL are different between normal smokers and non-smokers and in subjects with underlying lung disease (Daniele et al. 1985).

Bronchoalveolar lavage has been widely used as a research procedure, particularly in the investigation of interstitial lung disease, where it has provided a fascinating insight into the pathogenetic immune mechanisms underlying these disorders (Crystal et al. 1984). The location or locations within the lung, from which the bronchoalveolar cell population is derived, are not clear. Initial correlations between cell types in BAL and those seen in the pulmonary interstitium in lung biopsies have not been confirmed (Daniele et al. 1985). Instilled fluid will inevitably contact conducting airways between the tip of the bronchoscope and the alveolar wall, and cells lying superficially within these airways may be washed from the mucosal surface. About half of the fluid instilled is lost, presumably being held back long enough to be absorbed into the pulmonary circulation. It is difficult to envisage fluid instilled into a central airway, reaching alveoli in the lungs' periphery and returning to be aspirated again from that central airway. It is likely that most of the cells recovered are derived from the small airways of the lung. In support of this is the finding of large numbers of airway derived neutrophils in the bronchoalveolar population of even minor degrees of airway inflammation. The increases in neutrophils seen in smokers and the later stages of pulmonary sarcoidosis are also probably airway derived. Pathological studies in primate lung referred to earlier (Guerzon et al. 1979) have demonstrated a proportion of mast cells within the airway mucosa, increasing in number towards the lung periphery, and mast cells lying in the airway mucosa have also been demonstrated in asthmatic subjects (Cutz et al. 1978). It is estimated that a single segmental lavage contacts ten alveoli and associated conducting airways (Daniele et al. 1985). BAL therefore has the potential for recovering mast cells lying superficially in the bronchial mucosa and those free within the bronchial lumen. This population of mast cells being derived from a different site within the lung may possess distinct morphological and functional properties to those of dispersed human lung mast cells.

Morphological Heterogeneity of Human Lung Mast Cells

The clear anatomical distinction which exists for the gastrointestinal tract between mucosal mast cells in mucosal sites and connective tissue mast cells in connective tissues does not hold for lung. The majority of lung mast cells lie in perivascular or submucosal connective tissues. These cells contain granules which stain exclusively with alcian blue, like the mucosal mast cells of the intestinal tract, or may show varying degrees of safranin positivity. The proportions of the two types of cell vary greatly between different lung specimens. Similarly, in some specimens few mast cells can be identified after fixation in formol saline whereas in others mast cells in perivascular and submucosal connective tissues are well preserved. However, mast cells lying superficially in the airway mucosa and lamina propria stain exclusively with alcian blue and although well preserved after fixation in Carnoy's fluid they cannot be identified after fixation in formol saline (Flint et al. 1985b). Thus, whilst cells with the staining characteristics of either the classical connective tissue or mucosal type can be seen throughout the lung parenchyma, those in the mucosa appear to be mucosal in type. Similarly, mast cells identified in human bronchoalveolar lavage have the morphological properties of mucosal mast cells (Flint et al. 1985b). The heterogeneity seen in dispersed human lung mast cells has previously been described with respect to size (Schulman et al. 1982) and ultrastructure (Caulfield et al. 1980). The major type of dispersed lung mast cell has granules with crystalline contents (scrolls, lattices or gratings) which become amorphous on activation whilst other cells contain granules with an amorphous structure in the absence of stimulation. Dispersed lung mast cells vary in size and histamine content from 2 pg/cell in the smallest to 15 pg/cell in the largest. The response to fixation varies from preparation to preparation. In some, mast cells are well preserved in either fixative, whereas in others very few are preserved by formol saline.

It has not proved possible to differentiate two distinct subpopulations of human lung mast cells using monoclonal anti-mast cell antibodies and fluorescence or immunohistochemical techniques. Using several different monoclonal antibodies raised against human mastocytoma cell lines, Rimmer et al. (1984) were able to identify mast cells in both the mucosa and connective tissues of human gut or lung. Similarly, these antibodies will bind to both human bronchoalveolar and dispersed lung mast cells (Flint et al. 1985).

The underlying cause of these differences in staining reaction remains obscure. In the rat, they have been attributed to different glycosaminoglycans in the two cell types (Tas and Bernsden 1977) but this is unlikely to be the case from human lung where mast cells have been shown to be heparin containing (Metcalf et al. 1979). Similarly, although different lineages have been proposed in the rat (see Barrett and Metcalfe 1984) this seems unlikely in human lung where cells of both types lie in close proximity and there seems to be no sharp division to suggest two distinct subpopulations. Cells with the characteristics of staining and fixation of all degrees in between the two extremes can be seen. The answer perhaps lies in the early observation that the staining characteristics of embryonic mast cells of the rat shift from alcian blue to safranin positivity with maturity (Combs et al. 1965). Mast cells lying in exposed mucosal positions may never reach such a stage, undergoing constant challenge and degranulation. In connective tissue sites, however, there may be a gradual shift towards safranin positivity of the granules and resistance to formaldehyde fixation with time, perhaps due to a change in the glycosaminoglycan–protein matrix. This would explain the wide variations in the proportions of these mast cell types between lung specimens, which may depend upon the rate of formation and degranulation of mast cells. Alternatively mast cells may be influenced by factors present in the local microenvironment, to develop in different ways. Thus, factors present in the mucosa may lead to the development of "mucosal-type" characteristics, and those in connective tissues to the development of "connective tissue-type" characteristics. Either possibility would be consistent with the findings recently reported by Nakano et al. (1985) demonstrating a common precursor for both mucosal and connective tissue-type mast cells.

Human Lung Mast Cells

Human lung mast cells obtained in single cell suspensions using a combination of mechanical disruption and enzymic digestion (Paterson et al. 1976) have been shown, both ultrastructurally and on the basis of size and histamine release, to be heterogeneous. The major type of dispersed lung mast cell has granules with crystalline contents which become amorphous on activation, whilst other cells contain predominantly granules which have an amorphous structure in the absence of stimulation (Caulfield et al. 1980; Brinkman 1968). Partial purification of human lung mast cells after dispersion may be achieved by countercurrent centrifugal elutriation (Schulman et al. 1982). This technique separates cells according to size and density yielding mast cells of differing size and histamine content in different fractions and varying from 2 pg/cell in the smallest to 15 pg/cell in the largest (Schulman et al. 1983). They found these differences between the large and small cells extended to mediator release. The smaller cells respond poorly to IgE-mediated signals, releasing a lower percentage of histamine (and therefore a lower absolute amount) and less PGD_2.

Mediator Release from Human Bronchoalveolar Mast Cells

Mast cells have now been identified in human bronchoalveolar lavage, although estimates of the percentage of total cells that they comprise vary widely. In our own lavages mast cells ranged from 0.08%–3% (Flint et al. 1985) and in the bronchial lavages of Patterson and colleagues (Patterson et al. 1977) from 0.3%–0.7% with an identical mean histamine content per mast cell (1.0 pg/cell). Our group found a good correlation between mast cells and histamine content

(Fig. 3.1). Lower percentages have been identified by other groups (Tomioka et al. 1984; Agius et al. 1985). It is likely that such differences arise from differences in the lavage technique and subsequent processing of lavage fluid (Flint et al. 1985a). Small variations in technique can lead to considerable differences in differential cell counts (Mordelet-Dambrine et al. 1984). Another factor which may influence the percentage of bronchoalveolar mast cells is the underlying pathology of subjects undergoing lavage. Even at this early stage it is apparent that certain conditions are associated with an increase in the percentage of bronchoalveolar mast cells (Flint et al. 1985; Agius et al. 1985).

Human bronchoalveolar lavage contains a population of mast cells which are functionally competent. Unlike the early experiments utilising cells recovered by bronchial lavage (Patterson et al. 1977), the viability of cells recovered by BAL is good (80%–99%) and spontaneous rates of histamine release are low (usually <10%). In addition, bronchoalveolar mast cells will respond to an IgE-dependent challenge with histamine release that is dose (Fig. 3.2), time

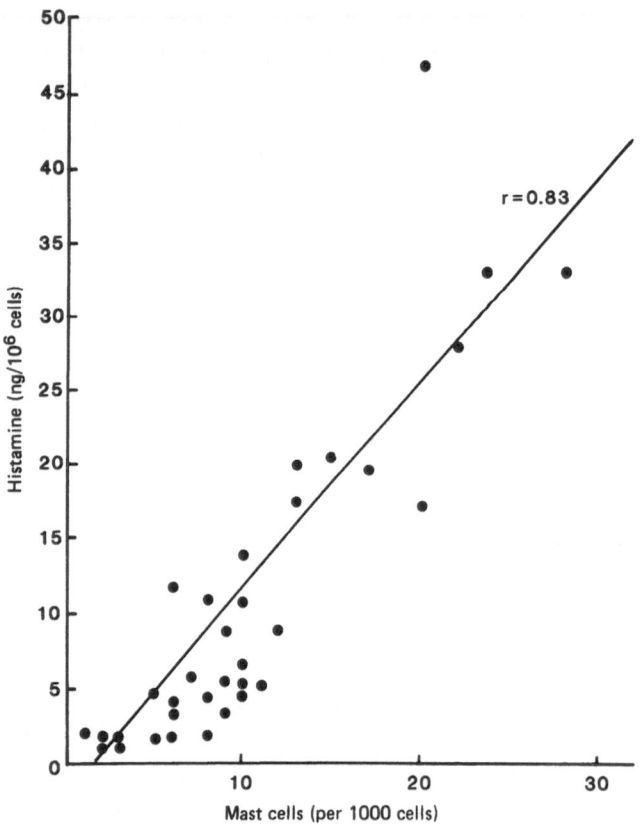

Fig. 3.1. The correlation between the histamine content of the bronchoalveolar cells and the percentage of mast cells.

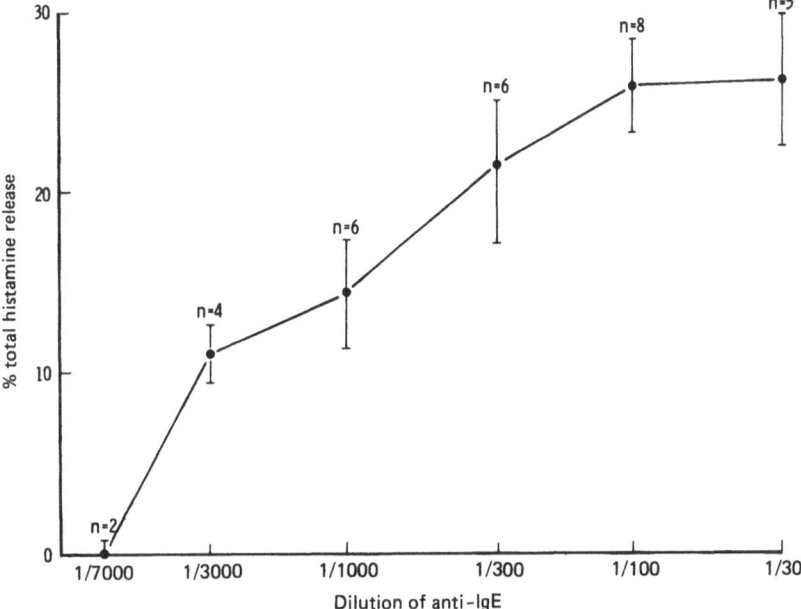

Fig. 3.2. Histamine release from human bronchoalveolar cells in response to anti-human IgE. Approximately 2×10^6 cells activated in a final volume of 250 ml. Points represent means (+ SEM) of the number of experiments.

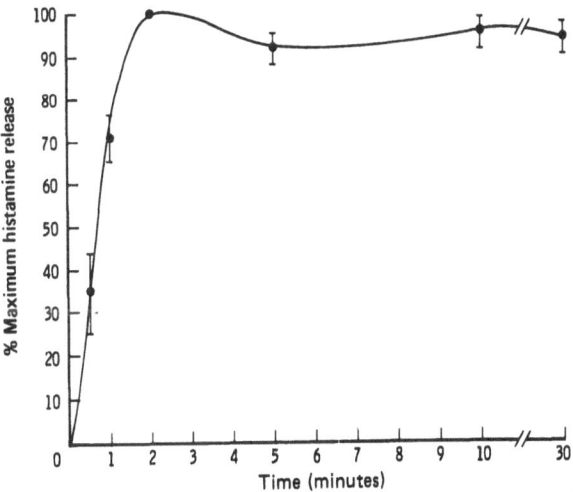

Fig. 3.3. Kinetics of IgE-dependent histamine release from human bronchoalveolar cells ($n=4$). Maximal release was $27.9 \pm 3.1\%$.

(Fig. 3.3) and energy-dependent (Flint et al. 1985b). Bronchoalveolar lavage recovers a mixed cell population including macrophages, lymphocytes, neutrophils and eosinophils.

Functioning IgE-Fc receptors have been identified on human lymphocytes and alveolar macrophages (Gonzales-Molina and Spiegelberg 1976; Capron et al. 1975), although these are of much lower affinity than those found on the mast cell surface. Nevertheless, no other human cell besides the mast cells and the basophil has yet been shown to contain and release histamine. It is therefore likely that the histamine containing cells within the bronchoalveolar cell population are mast cells and that IgE-dependent histamine release follows mast cell activation. This is supported by the direct correlation between the mast cell number and the histamine content of the bronchoalveolar cell population. It remains possible, however, that mast cell histamine release is influenced by the presence of other cell types within the lavage population.

A typical lavage contains no red cells. Nevertheless, the possibility that the histamine containing cells within the lavage are blood basophils which have migrated into the lung must be considered. Although of a similar size with similar affinity for cationic dyes, bronchoalveolar mast cells appear morphologically distinct. In particular the nucleus is typically oval and eccentric rather than segmented. The functional profile of these two histamine containing cell populations is also quite different. The response to IgE-dependent challenge differs significantly between peripheral blood basophils and bronchoalveolar cells, even in the same subjects, both in the magnitude of response at different

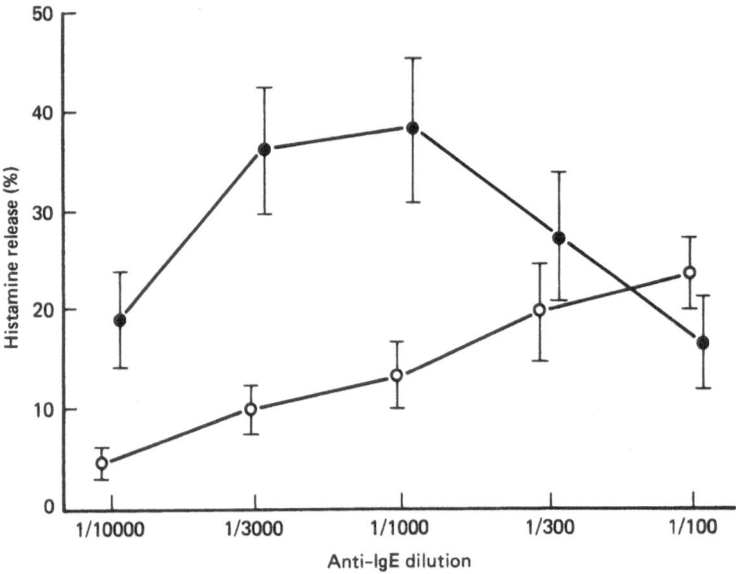

Fig. 3.4. Histamine release from human bronchoalveolar cells (○) and peripheral blood leucocytes (●); $n=6$.

dilutions of anti-IgE and in the speed of this response (Fig. 3.4). Histamine release from peripheral basophils is much slower than from bronchoalveolar or dispersed lung cells (Leung et al. 1986). Finally, unlike bronchoalveolar cells, histamine release from basophils is not inhibited by DSCG or salbutamol.

Thus human bronchoalveolar lavage provides an alternative in vitro model of human mast cell function. The bronchoalveolar mast cell preparation has several advantages over human dispersed lung mast cells. Firstly, bronchoalveolar mast cells are not subject to mechanical or enzymic trauma unlike dispersed lung mast cells, nor do they require passive sensitisation prior to challenge. Their responses may therefore more closely resemble the events occurring in vivo. Secondly, human lung cells are dispersed from lung tissue resected at thoracotomy. They are therefore almost invariably derived from heavy smokers with an underlying bronchial carcinoma and dispersed from tissue adjacent to tumour. It is possible that this may lead to an alteration in their functional characteristics. Human bronchoalveolar mast cells can be obtained by lavage from patients with widely differing underlying pathologies. There is thus the potential for studying mast cell function in different pathological conditions. Thirdly, lying superficially within the lung, the study of bronchoalveolar mast cells may be more relevant to the events that follow the inhalation of antigen in asthmatic subjects.

References

Agius RM, Godfrey RC, Holgate ST (1985) Mast cell and histamine content of human bronchoalveolar lavage. Thorax 40: 760–767

Barrett KE, Metcalfe DD (1984) Mast cell heterogeneity: evidence and implications. J Clin Immunol 4: 253–261

Brinkman L (1968) The mast cell in normal human bronchus and lung. J Ultrastruct Res 23: 115–123

Capron A, Dessaint JO, Capron M, Bazin H (1975) Specific IgE antibodies in immune adherence of normal macrophages to *Schistosoma mansoni* schistosomules. Nature 253: 474–475

Caulfield JP, Lewis RA, Hein A, Austen KF (1980) Secretion in dissociated human pulmonary mast cells. Evidence for solubilisation of granule contents before discharge. J Cell Biol 85: 299–312

Combs JW, Lagunoff D, Benditt EP (1965) Differentiation and proliferation of the embryonic mast cells of the rat. J Cell Biol 25: 577–592

Crystal RG, Bitterman PB, Rennard SI, Hance AJ, Keogh BA (1984) Interstitial lung disease of unknown cause. N Engl J Med 310: 154–166

Crystal RG, Reynolds HY, Kalica AR (1986) Bronchoalveolar lavage. The report of an international conference. Chest 89: 122–131

Cutz E, Lewison H, Cooper DM (1978) Ultrastructure of airways in children with asthma. Histopathol 2: 407–421

Daniele RP, Elias JA, Epstein PE, Rossman MD (1985) Bronchoalveolar lavage: role in the pathogenesis, diagnosis and management of interstitial lung disease. Ann Int Med 102: 93–108

Findlay SR, Strotsky E, Luterman K, Hernady Z, Ohman JL (1983) Allergens detected in association with airborne particles capable of penetrating into the periphery of the lung. Am Rev Resp Dis 128: 1008–1012

Flint KC, Leung KBP, Hudspith BN, Brostoff J, Johnson NMcI (1985a) Bronchoalveolar mast cells in extrinsic asthma. Brit Med J (Letter) 291: 1354

Flint KC, Leung KBP, Pearce FL, Hudspith BN, Brostoff J, Johnson NMcI (1985b) Human mast cells recovered by bronchoalveolar lavage: their morphology, histamine release and the effects of sodium cromoglycate. Clin Sci 68: 427–432

Flint KC, Hudspith BN, Leung KBP et al. (1986) Bronchoalveolar mast cells in sarcoidosis: increased numbers and accentuation of histamine release. Thorax 41: 94–98

Floyer J (1698) A treatise of the asthma. R Wilkin, London. Quoted by Sakula A. Sir John Floyer's A treatise of the asthma. Thorax 1984; 39: 248–254

Gonzales-Molina A, Spiegelberg HL (1976) Binding of IgE myeloma proteins to human cultured lymphoblastoid cells. J Immunol 117: 1836–1845

Guerzon GM, Pare PD, Michoud MC, Hogg JC (1979) The number and distribution of mast cells in monkey lungs. Am Rev Resp Dis 119: 59–66

Hogg JC, Pare PD, Boucher RC, Michoud MC, Guerzon G, Moroz L (1977) Pathologic abnormalities in asthma. In: Lichtenstein LM, Austen KF (eds) Asthma II. Physiology, immunopharmacology and treatment, 2nd International symposium. Academic Press, New York, pp 1–14

Leung KBP, Flint KC, Brostoff J, Hudspith BN, Johnson NMcI, Pearce FL (1986) Some properties of mast cells obtained by bronchoalveolar lavage. Agents and Actions 18: 100–112

Metcalfe DD, Lewis RA, Silbert JE, Rosenberg RD, Wasserman SI, Austen KF (1979) Isolation and characteristics of heparin from human lung. J Clin Invest 64: 1537–1543

Mordelet-Dambrine M, Arnoux A, Stanislas-Le Guern G, Sandron D, Chretien J, Huchon G (1984) Processing of lung lavage fluid causes variability in the bronchoalveolar cell count. Am Rev Resp Dis 130: 305–306

Nakano T, Sonoda T, Hayashi C et al. (1985) Fate of bone marrow-derived cultured mast cells after intracutaneous, intraperitoneal and intravenous transfer into genetically mast cell deficient W/Wv mice. J Exp Med 162: 1025–1043

Paterson NAM, Wasserman SI, Said JW, Austen KF (1976) Release of chemical mediators from partially purified human lung mast cells. J Immunol 117: 1356–1362

Patterson R, Tomita Y, Oh SH, Suszko IM, Pruzansky JJ (1974) Respiratory mast cells and basophil cells. Clin Exp Immunol 16: 223–226

Patterson R, McKenna JM, Suszko IM et al. (1977) Living histamine containing cells from the bronchial lumen of humans. Description and comparison of histamine content with cells of the rhesus monkey. J Clin Invest 59: 217–225

Patterson R, Suszko IM, Harris KE (1978) The in vivo transfer of antigen-induced airway reactions by bronchial lumen mast cells. J Clin Invest 62: 519–524

Peters SP, Schulman ES, Schleimer RP, MacGlashan DW, Newball HH, Lichtenstein LM (1982) Dispersed human lung mast cells. Pharmacologic aspects and comparison with human lung tissue fragments. Am Rev Resp Dis 126: 1034–1039

Reynolds HY, Newball HH (1974) Analysis of proteins and respiratory cells from human lung by bronchial lavage. J Lab Clin Med 84: 559–579

Rimmer ER, Tuberville C, Horton MA (1984) Human mast cells detected by monoclonal antibodies. J Clin Pathol 37: 1249–1255

Salvato G (1968) Some histological changes in chronic bronchitis and asthma. Thorax 23: 168–172

Schulman ES, MacGlashan DW, Peters SP, Schleimer RP, Newball H, Lichtenstein LM (1982) Human lung mast cells: purification and characterisation. J Immunol 129: 2662–2667

Schulman ES, Kagey-Sabotka A, MacGlashan DW et al. (1983) Heterogeneity of human lung mast cells. J Immunol 131: 1936–1941

Simani AS, Inoue S, Hogg JC (1974) Penetration of respiratory epithelium of guinea pigs following exposure to cigarette smoke. Lab Invest 31: 75–78

Tas J, Bernsden RG (1977) Does heparin occur in mucosal mast cells of the rat small intestine? J Histochem Cytochem 25: 1058–1062

Tomioka M, Ida S, Shindoh Y, Ishihara T, Takishima T (1984) Mast cells in the bronchoalveolar lumen of patients with bronchial asthma. Am Rev Resp Dis 129: 1000–1005

Some Functional Properties of Human Bronchoalveolar and Dispersed Lung Mast Cells

Introduction

Much of our knowledge of mast cell function stems from early work with rodent cells, usually those harvested from the rat peritoneal cavity. In the light of the now considerable evidence of heterogeneity of mast cell function between different species, this work must be interpreted with great caution. The challenge of human lung fragments via IgE-dependent mechanisms in vitro is one step closer to human disease. However, activation of lung fragments will include effects on vascular tissue and lung parenchyma in addition to bronchi. The activation of such a mixed population of cells produces results that are very variable (Church and Young 1983) and the contribution of any single cell type to the response of the intact tissue is impossible to define. Dispersion of free cells from lung fragments allows the study of the function of mast cells in isolated cell suspensions, and ultimately with the purification of mast cells, their function in isolation. However, with increasing evidence of heterogeneity of mast cell function even between mast cells from different sites in the same tissue (Pearce 1982), the response of mast cells dispersed from the lung parenchyma may not be relevant to events occurring at the mucosal surface. Thus mast cells in bronchoalveolar lavage may possess functional properties that are distinct from those in dispersed cell preparations. In direct comparisons between these two preparations differences and similarities are now being defined.

Histamine Content and IgE-Dependent Histamine Release

The histamine content of human dispersed lung mast cells is very variable and heavily dependent upon cell size (Schulman et al. 1983). The mean histamine content in different studies varies from 2–15 pg/cell. In bronchoalveolar lavage, I found values for the mast cell histamine content have varied from 1–3 pg/cell. When mast cells are identified by alcian blue–safranin staining and lysed directly with perchloric acid the value for the histamine content of bronchoalveolar mast cells differs significantly from that of dispersed lung mast cells (1.0±0.1 vs 2.6±0.4, $P<0.001$, Flint et al. 1985).

A common property of all mast cells is their capacity to release histamine in response to IgE-dependent activation. However, the magnitude of that response may vary considerably, depending upon the occupancy of cell surface IgE-Fc receptors and the sensitivity of receptor response coupling. Human dispersed lung cells rarely release significant amounts of histamine in response to challenge with anti-IgE unless they are first passively sensitised (Fig. 4.1). In contrast, human bronchoalveolar cells respond reliably to anti-IgE challenge with histamine release without the need for passive sensitisation (Leung et al. 1986). This initial lack of response by dispersed lung cells does not seem to be the result of the dispersion process itself. It is not due to incubation with proteolytic enzymes during enzymic dispersion as both mechanically and enzymically dispersed preparations behave in the same way. Furthermore, undispersed human lung fragments also require passive sensitisation for significant mediaor release (Young and Church 1983) and passive sensitisation of lung fragments

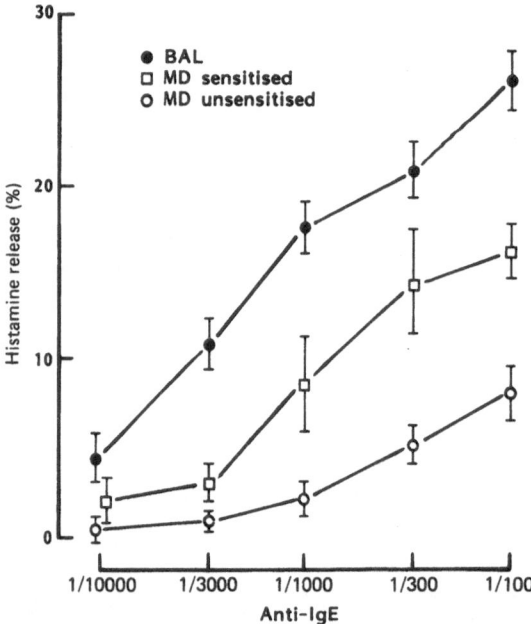

Fig. 4.1. Anti-IgE induced histamine release from enzymatically dispersed human lung cells either before (○) or after (□) passive sensitisation ($n=6$) and from human bronchoalveolar cells (●, $n=6$, non-passively sensitised). *Points* represent means with SE bars.

prior to full enzymic dispersion is as effective as passive sensitisation after dispersion (Leung et al. 1986).

Histamine release from dispersed human lung cells can be increased to the same level as bronchoalveolar cells by passive sensitisation, suggesting that the difference in the degree of histamine release may be due to differences in the occupancy of mast cell IgE-Fc receptors. Bronchoalveolar mast cells are sensitised in vivo, and retain their capacity to respond to IgE-dependent stimuli in vitro. IgE secreting plasma cells have been identified in BAL (Lawrence et al. 1978) and significant levels of IgE have been detected in human lung lining fluid (Merrill et al. 1980). This may contribute to the in vivo sensitisation of mast cells lying superficially. An alternative possibility is that there is a difference in the sensitivity of receptor-response coupling between the two mast cell populations and further experiments are required to distinguish between these two possibilities.

The Effect of Anti-allergic Compounds

Disodium Cromoglycate

Disodium cromoglycate (DSCG) is an effective anti-allergic compound in clinical practice (Silverman et al. 1972). It is a potent inhibitor of anaphylactic histamine release from rat peritoneal mast cells (Orr 1977) but paradoxically is ineffective against IgE-dependent histamine release from human lung fragments (Church and Young 1983; Butchers et al. 1979) and human dispersed lung mast cells (Church et al. 1983). Many other drugs with greater potency than cromoglycate on rat mast cells have failed to exhibit clinical efficacy in asthmatics in vivo (Stokes and Morley 1981). In addition to reports of the prophylactic effect of DSCG against a variety of non-immunologic stimuli to bronchoconstriction, these observations have led to speculation that the mode of action of DSCG in vivo may not be related to its mast cell stabilising properties. However, anti-allergic compounds inhibit histamine release from mast cells from different species and different tissues to differing extents (Pearce 1982) and the finding that DSCG is a significantly better inhibitor of IgE-dependent histamine release from human bronchoalveolar mast cells than from human dispersed lung mast cells may provide an explanation for the clinical efficacy of this drug (Fig. 4.2). Even when challenged with optimal concentrations of anti-IgE, histamine release from human bronchoalveolar cells was significantly inhibited (Flint et al. 1985).

In parallel experiments, the anti-allergic effect of DSCG on human bronchoalveolar and human dispersed lung has now been investigated (Leung et al. 1986). A major difference is the marked tachyphylaxis shown by this drug in its effect on dispersed lung mast cells. After 10 min its activity is greatly reduced

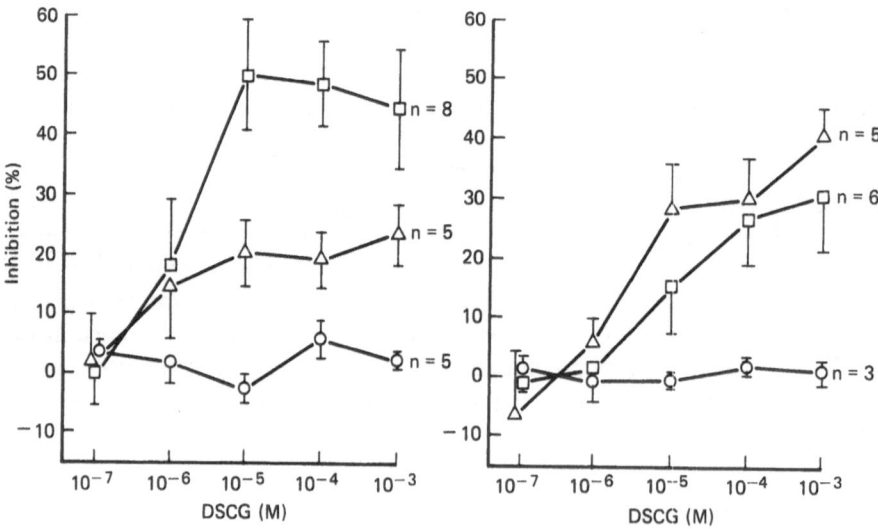

Fig. 4.2. Effect of DSCG (**a**) with 10 min pre-incubation and (**b**) with no pre-incubation, on anti-IgE induced histamine release from basophils (O), BAL mast cells (□) and dispersed lung cells (△). Values are means ± SEM for the number (*n*) of experiments noted.

and after 30 min is negligible (Church et al. 1983; Leung et al. 1986). In contrast the activity of DSCG on bronchoalveolar mast cells increases after 10 min preincubation and it is at this preincubation time that the difference between its effect on the two mast cell preparations is most marked (Leung et al. 1986). The latter finding is more in keeping with the prophylactic effect of DSCG in vivo. Allergen challenge in vivo is unlikely to be optimal for mast cell activation and at low levels of activation, inhibition of mediator release by anti-allergic compounds such as DSCG is likely to be more effective.

The tissue and species selectivity in the extent to which mast cell histamine release is inhibited by anti-allergic compounds (Pearce 1982) has led to great difficulty in the attempts of the pharmaceutical industry to develop appropriate in vitro models for the screening of these drugs (Stokes and Morley 1981; Church 1978). The rat peritoneal mast cell has been used for this purpose for many years but with little success in predicting in vivo efficacy. A preparation of human lung mast cells is obviously more appropriate but it is now apparent that these are also heterogeneous in their response to anti-allergic compounds. Lying superficially within the lung, bronchoalveolar mast cells would be readily available to inhaled antigen and mediators released as a result of such antigen contact would be released directly onto the airway surface. These cells would therefore be in an ideal position to provide the initial interaction with inhaled antigen. Studies of the functional profile of these cells would therefore be more relevant to the events that occur after antigen inhalation in vivo and they could provide a more appropriate model for the in vitro screening of anti-allergic compounds.

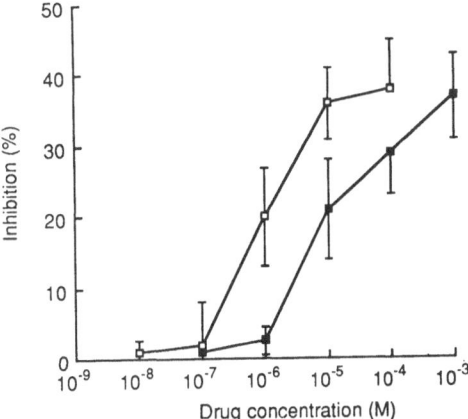

Fig. 4.3. Inhibition of histamine release from mast cells isolated from human dispersed lung by sodium cromoglycate (■) and nedocromil sodium (□). The drugs were added at the same time as the anti-IgE. Results are expressed as mean ± SE.

Nedocromil Sodium

This drug is of interest in this respect as it is a novel anti-allergic compound developed for use in bronchial asthma. It is an effective inhibitor of anaphylactic histamine release from both rat peritoneal mast cells and the rat intestinal mucosal mast cell (TSC Orr, personal communication). Preliminary results suggest that nedocromil sodium is an effective prophylactic of exercise-induced asthma and in therapeutic clinical use (Lal et al. 1985). Nedocromil sodium gave a similar maximum suppression of histamine release as DSCG but was more active on a molar basis when tested on dispersed human lung mast cells (Fig. 4.3). Against bronchoalveolar lavage mast cells it gave greater maximum suppression and was more active on a molar basis than DSCG (Fig. 4.4). Its anti-allergic effect shows considerable tachyphylaxis at 10 min against histamine release from human dispersed lung mast cells (Leung et al. 1986) and after 10 min preincubation its activity on IgE-dependent histamine release from human bronchoalveolar mast cells is significantly greater than from human dispersed lung mast cells (Fig. 4.5).

Salbutamol

Salbutamol is an effective beta-2 receptor agonist which is widely prescribed because of its relaxant effect on bronchial smooth muscle. It has little effect on anaphylactic histamine release from rat peritoneal mast cells (Johnson and Moran 1970) but inhibits histamine release from human lung fragments (Church and Young 1983) and dispersed human lung mast cells (Church et al. 1983). The anti-allergic activity of salbutamol on human dispersed lung mast cells shows no

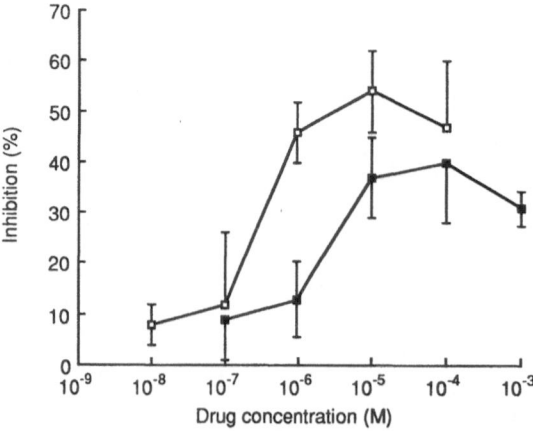

Fig. 4.4. Inhibition of histamine release from bronchoalveolar mast cells by sodium cromoglycate (■) and nedocromil sodium (□). The drugs were added at the time of anti-IgE stimulation. Results are expressed as mean ± SE.

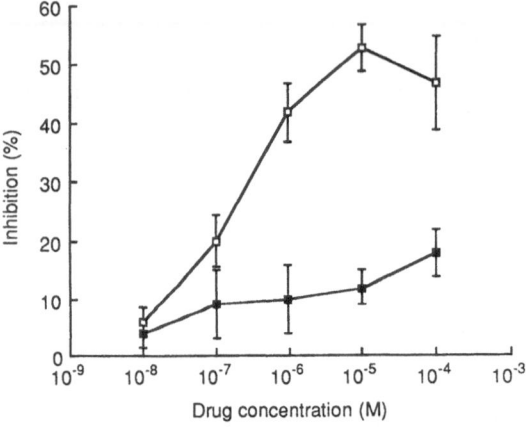

Fig. 4.5. Inhibition by nedocromil sodium of anti-IgE induced histamine release from bronchoal-veolar mast cells (□) and dispersed mast cells (■). Effect of pre-incubating the cells for 10 min before challenge with anti-IgE. Results are expressed as mean ± SE.

significant tachyphylaxis after 10 min preincubation. This drug is a highly significant inhibitor of IgE-dependent histamine release from human bronchoal-veolar mast cells (Leung et al. 1986). Because of its bronchodilator effect it is difficult to demonstrate a prophylactic anti-allergic action of salbutamol in vivo. However, in subjects with hay fever, a related beta-2 agonist, fenoterol, has been shown to inhibit the direct response to allergen challenge (Schumacker 1980; Borum and Mygind 1980). As its only other effect in the nose is to dilate blood vessels it is likely that this inhibition is due to its anti-allergic properties with inhibition of mast cell mediator release. In addition, in asthmatic subjects, systemic beta-2 agonists shift the dose-response curve for the appearance of histamine and neutrophil chemotactic factor in peripheral blood after antigen challenge suggesting inhibition of mediator release in vivo (Martin et al. 1980).

Theophylline

Theophylline is a potent inhibitor of anaphylactic histamine release from the connective tissue mast cell of the rat but is almost entirely inactive against histamine release from rodent mucosal mast cells. More recently it has been shown to inhibit IgE-dependent histamine release from human lung fragments in vitro. This compound also shows significant anti-allergic activity against both human bronchoalveolar and human dispersed lung mast cells. Whilst this is the only drug tested to achieve almost 100% inhibition of anti-IgE induced histamine release, this occurred only at high concentrations (10 mM). At low concentrations approaching those that might be achieved in vivo, this drug had little activity.

In summary, there are functional differences between human bronchoalveolar and human dispersed lung mast cells, both in the magnitude of their response to anti-IgE and in their response to the anti-allergic drugs. It is difficult to know how fundamental these differences are. They appear to represent differences in degree rather than differences in absolute reactivity. Thus IgE-dependent histamine release from human dispersed lung mast cells can be increased to the same level as bronchoalveolar mast cells by passive sensitisation. Furthermore, the response of both preparations to salbutamol and theophylline is similar, as is the response to nedocromil sodium and DSCG, without preincubation. The major difference arises when nedocromil or DSCG are preincubated with dispersed lung or bronchoalveolar cells. The differences observed may be the result of trauma to mast cells occurring during their dispersion from lung fragments rather than the result of ontogenically distinct mast cell subpopulations within the lung. This interpretation of these functional studies would be in keeping with the results of the morphological studies, where there was no clear distinction between the two preparations morphologically. Whatever the cause of such differences the human bronchoalveolar mast cell preparation would seem to be a more appropriate in vitro model of human mast cell function.

References

Borum P, Mygind N (1980) Inhibition of the immediate reaction in the nose by the beta-2 adrenostimulant fenoterol. J Allergy Clin Immunol 66: 25–32
Butchers PR, Fullarton JR, Skidmore IF, Thompson LE, Varday J, Wheeldon A (1979) A comparison of the anti-anaphylactic activities of salbutamol and disodium cromoglycate in the rat, the rat mast cell and in human lung tissue. Br J Pharmacol 67: 23–32
Church MK (1978) Cromoglycate-like anti-allergic drugs: a review. Drugs Today 14: 281–341

Church MK, Young KD (1983) The characteristics of histamine release from human lung fragments by sodium cromoglycate, salbutamol and chlorpromazine. Br J Pharmacol 78: 671–679

Church MK, Holgate ST, Pao GJK (1983) Histamine release from mechanically and enzymatically dispersed human lung mast cells: inhibition by salbutamol and cromoglycate. Br J Pharmacol 79: 347p

Flint KC, Leung KBP, Pearce FL, Hudspith BN, Brostoff J, Johnson NMcI (1985) Human mast cells recovered by bronchoalveolar lavage: their morphology, histamine release and the effects of sodium cromoglycate. Clin Sci 68: 427–432

Johnson AR, Moran NC (1970) Inhibition of the release of histamine from rat mast cells: the effects of cold and adrenergic drugs on the release of histamine by 48/80 and antigen. J Pharmacol Exp Ther 175: 632–640

Lal S, Malhotra S, Gribben S, Hodder D (1985) Nedocromil sodium: a new drug for the management of bronchial asthma. Thorax 39: 809–812

Lawrence EC, Blaese RM, Martin RR, Stevens PM (1978) Immunoglobulin secreting cells in normal human bronchial lavage fluids. J Clin Invest 62: 832–835

Law D, Jackson L, Fulmer J (1982) Bronchoalveolar lavage analysis in the interstitial lung diseases. Am Rev Resp Dis 125: 105–108

Leung KBP, Flint KC, Brostoff J, Hudspith BN, Johnson NMcI, Pearce FL (1986) Some properties of mast cells obtained by human bronchoalveolar lavage. Agents and Actions 18: 100–112

Martin AL, Atkins PC, Dunsky PH, Zweiman B (1980) The effect of theophylline, terbutaline and prednisolone upon antigen-induced bronchospasm and mediator release. J Allergy Clin Immunol 68: 286–289

Merrill WW, Naegel GP, Reynolds HY (1980) Analysis of normal human bronchoalveolar lavage fluid IgE and comparison to immunoglobulins G and A. J Lab Clin Med 94: 494–500

Orr TSC (1977) Mode of action of disodium cromoglycate. Acta Allergologica (Suppl 13) 32: 9–27

Pearce FL (1982) Functional heterogeneity of mast cells from different species and tissues. Klin Wschr 60: 954–957

Schulman ES, Kagey-Sabotka A, MacGlashan DW et al. (1983) Heterogeneity of human lung mast cells. J Immunol 131: 1936–1941

Schumacker NJ (1980) Effect of a beta-adrenergic agonist, fenoterol, on nasal sensitivity to allergen. J Allergy Clin Immunol 66: 33–37

Silverman M, Connolly NM, Balfour-Lynn L, Godfrey S (1972) Long term trial of disodium cromoglycate and isoprenaline in children with asthma. Br Med J 3: 378–381

Stokes TC, Morley J (1981) Prospects for an oral intal. Br J Dis Chest 75: 1–14

Young KD, Church MK (1983) Passive anaphylaxis in human lung fragments as a model for testing anti-allergic drugs: its variability and constraints. Int Arch Allergy Appl Immunol

Hyperosmolar Histamine Release from Human Lung Mast Cells: Its Relevance to Exercise-Induced Asthma

Introduction

Sir John Floyer (1698) was the first to remark that "all violent exercise makes the asthmatic to breathe short". After an initial bronchodilation which persists for the duration of the exercise, breathlessness increases as the asthmatic bronchoconstricts reaching peak in severity at 3–5 min (Herxheimer 1946). The severity of the post-exercise bronchoconstriction increases with increasing duration and work load to reach a maximum after 6–8 min of exercise at 70% of maximum oxygen uptake (Silverman and Anderson 1972). Prolonging the duration of exercise or repeating the exercise within 3 h (the refractory period) results in a reduction in the severity of post-exercise bronchoconstriction (Godfrey et al. 1973; Edmunds et al. 1978).

The observation that at equivalent work loads swimming was less asthmagenic than running led to studies to examine the effect of the conditioning of inspired air on the severity of exercise-induced bronchoconstriction. Several authors made the observation that exercising whilst breathing humid air lessened the severity of exercise-induced asthma (Weinstein et al. 1976; Chen and Horton 1977; Barr-Orr et al. 1977). Further studies showed that exercising whilst breathing cold dry air increased the severity of exercise-induced asthma (Strauss et al. 1977) whilst air preconditioned to body temperature and humidity abolished the subsequent fall in forced expiratory volume in one second (FEV) (Strauss et al. 1978). Finally, isocapnic hyperventilation was found to be capable of provoking as much asthma as exercise (Deal et al. 1979a). In all of these conditions there was a good general correlation between provoked asthma and respiratory heat loss leading to the hypothesis that the initiating event was respiratory heat loss which resulted in airways cooling (Deal et al. 1979b). Events responsible for the second reaction sequence linking airways cooling to bronchoconstriction remained obscure. Their failure to find neutrophil chemotactic factor in the serum despite significant bronchoconstriction or to find a refractory period after hyperventilation-induced asthma (Deal et al. 1980; Stearns et al. 1981) led these authors to propose that a neural reflex was most likely and that the refractory period after exercise was probably due to catecholamine release.

There is, however, mounting evidence that the release of chemical mediators may be of major importance in exercise-induced asthma. Measurements of oesophageal temperature (Deal et al. 1979c) and detailed thermal mapping of the human respiratory tract (McFadden et al. 1983) confirm that falls in temperature do occur during hyperventilation. During quiet breathing most warming and humidification occurs in the upper respiratory tract but with increasing ventilation and decreasing temperature this zone passes deeper into the lung periphery. With large amounts of frigid air the tracheal temperature may fall as low as 19–20°C and in the right lower lobe may reach the mid–20°C's (McFadden et al. 1982; McFadden et al. 1983). However, the change in lung functions lags considerably behind the fall in temperature which returns to normal within a few seconds of exercise whilst airflow obstruction progressively worsens to reach a peak at 5–10 min and slowly abates over 30–60 min (Herxheimer 1946). This behaviour would be quite unlike that of a neural reflex and is more in keeping with the release of a chemical mediator. Further evidence in support of mediator release in the evolution of post-exercise bronchoconstriction comes from several sources. Disodium cromoglycate is an effective prophylactic of exercise-induced asthma (Davies 1968) and although this drug has other properties its activity in vivo has never been shown conclusively to be due to anything other than the inhibition of mast cell mediator release. Furthermore, both histamine and neutrophil chemotactic factor have been detected in peripheral blood in increased concentrations during exercise-induced bronchoconstriction and both the increase in serum mediators and the changes in pulmonary mechanics are inhibited by disodium cromoglycate (Lee et al. 1982). In this study, post-exercise basophilia, an alternative explanation for the rise in plasma histamine, occurred equally in controls and asthmatics with or without exercise-induced asthma but significant elevations in plasma histamine occurred only in those with post-exercise bronchoconstriction. An elevation of plasma histamine has also been detected during isocapnic hyperventilation induced asthma (Nagakura et al. 1983) although without a simultaneous increase in neutrophil chemotactic activity. The detection of an elevation of the latter after exercise but not after hyperventilation challenge may be the result of changes in the pulmonary circulation on exercise leading to greater washout of this high molecular weight factor. Histamine is a considerably smaller molecule. It has also been established that hyperventilation is capable of rendering subjects refractory to exercise and exercise of rendering these patients refractory to hyperventilation (Bar-Yishay et al. 1983). The underlying mechanism of this refractoriness is not fully explained but it has been suggested that it is due to depletion of stored mediators. In support of this is the finding that exercise may render subjects refractory to doses of antigen that previously caused broncho-constriction (Weiller-Ravell and Godfrey 1981), suggesting that the two forms of challenge utilise the same pathway. Experimental evidence to date would therefore be compatible with the concept of mediator depletion.

It is doubtful that heat loss can be regarded as the sole trigger of exercise-induced asthma. More recently, it has become apparent that the general correlation between respiratory heat loss and subsequent bronchoconstriction is not absolute. Running whilst breathing dry or humid air causes more post-exertional bronchoconstriction than swimming despite identical levels of respiratory heat loss (Bar-Yishay et al. 1982) and exercising whilst breathing hot dry air may induce bronchoconstriction without any evidence of airways cooling (Anderson et al. 1983). The relationship between temperature and humidity in the conditioning of inspired air is complex as temperature changes are inextricably linked to water loss. As the temperature of air rises its capacity to hold water increases and it is humidified by evaporation from the airway lining. There is a consequent increase in the osmolarity of the airway lining fluid in addition to airway cooling due to the latent heat of evaporation. Bronchocons-triction by hot air in absence of airway cooling (Anderson et al. 1983) suggests that changes in osmolarity per se can result in bronchoconstriction. The process of humidification accounts for the vast majority of the total heat transferred (McFadden et al. 1984) and this may in part explain the observed relationship between respiratory heat exchange and exercise-induced asthma.

Mannitol-Induced Histamine Release

Further evidence that changes in osmolarity in isolation may result in bronchoconstriction is provided by studies of the effects of nebulised hypertonic solutions in asthmatic subjects. The inhalation of hyperosmolar solutions of saline or of sucrose will result in bronchoconstriction (Schoeffel et al. 1981; Smith and Anderson 1986).

Basophils

Hyperosmolar release of histamine from human basophils has been previously demonstrated (Findlay et al. 1981). Increasing concentrations of mannitol from 0.1–1.0 M (final osmolarities of 360–1270 mosm/kg) caused a dose-dependent release of histamine reaching an optimum of 50% at 0.75 M. This release was felt to be neither toxic nor lytic. It did not occur at 4°C and was inhibited at concentrations of mannitol greater than 0.75 M. Histamine release was blocked by inhibitors of phospholipid metabolism, was partially inhibited by EDTA and was associated with minimal release of lactic dehydrogenase. In addition, electron microscopic studies demonstrated features characteristic of specific degranulation rather than cell lysis.

The mechanism of such mediator release in response to hyperosmolar challenge is independent of those involving the IgE receptor as desensitisation to anti-IgE induced histamine release did not inhibit subsequent hyperosmolar challenge. As both processes are inhibited by p-bromphenacylbromide and eicosa-5,8,11,14-tetraenoic acid, it can be speculated that both processes require the formation of one or more phospholipid intermediates. The hyperosmolar release process is similar in many respects to release induced by the phorbol diester TPA (Findlay et al. 1981; Hook and Siraganian 1981). Both are only partially dependent on extracellular calcium, are not inhibited by cyclic adenosine monophosphate (cAMP) active drugs and are enhanced in cells desensitised to anti-IgE (Schleimer et al. 1981). It has been suggested that TPA might mobilise calcium from intracellular reservoirs (Smith and Iden 1979) and so a similar mechanism might be involved in hyperosmolar challenge.

Lung Mast Cells

Histamine release from human dispersed lung mast cells has also been demonstrated in response to increasing concentrations of mannitol (Eggleston et al. 1984). Mannitol induced the release of histamine in a dose-dependent manner with a maximal release of 11.9% at 0.75 M, lower than that observed from basophils.

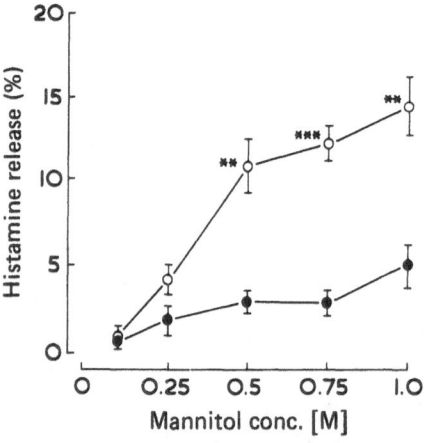

Fig. 5.1. Mannitol-induced histamine release from human bronchoalveolar (○, $n=28$) and dispersed lung cells (●, $n=7$). Approximately 2×10^6 cells challenged in Tyrodes buffer (final volume 200 μl) and the reaction allowed to proceed for 10 min. *Points* represent means and SEM.

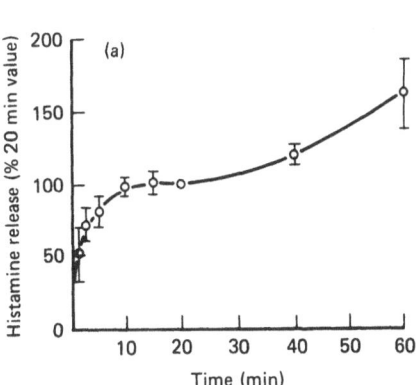
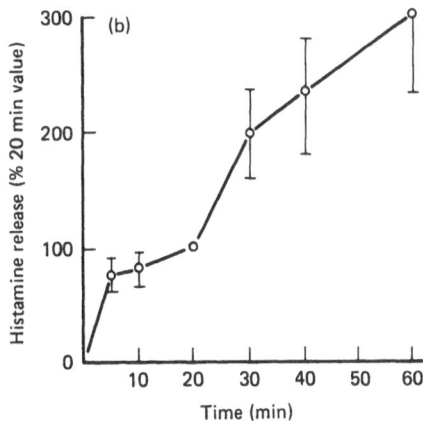

Fig. 5.2. The kinetics of mannitol-induced (0.75 M) release from **a** human bronchoalveolar cells and **b** human dispersed lung cells. Release has been standardised to 100% at 20 min, net histamine release at 20 min being 16.7%±3.0% of total cellular histamine for bronchoalveolar cells and 4.2%±1.0% (mean ± SE) for dispersed lung. Sixty-minute values were 23.8%±7.6% for bronchoalveolar cells and 12.1%±2.5% net histamine release for dispersed lung cells (142% and 288% of the 20-min values respectively).

Challenge of both human bronchoalveolar and human dispersed lung mast cells with increasing extracellular concentrations of mannitol results in a dose-dependent release of histamine (Fig. 5.1). Mannitol-induced histamine release from human bronchoalveolar cells was significantly greater than spontaneous histamine release at concentrations from 0.25–1.0 M and was a rapid process, achieving 50% of its 20 min value within 1 min and 80% within 5 min.

Histamine release from human dispersed lung mast cells in response to challenge with mannitol is slower. At 10 min, mannitol-induced histamine release from human dispersed lung mast cells is greatly below that of human bronchoalveolar cells at all mannitol concentrations (Fig. 5.2). Net histamine release from dispersed lung cells in response to challenge with 0.75 M mannitol reached only 3% at 10 min compared with 12.5% net release from bronchoalveolar cells.

At 40 min mannitol-induced histamine release from dispersed lung cells achieved similar levels to those reported by Eggleston et al. (1984) but in the experiments reported here histamine release continued to increase with mannitol concentration up to 1.0 M with no descending limb to the dose-response curve. It is therefore difficult to support the conclusion of Eggleston et al. (1984) that mannitol-induced histamine release from human dispersed lung mast cells is not, at least in part, a lytic process. The kinetics of this process show a small initial increase (Fig. 5.2) but then mannitol-induced histamine release from dispersed lung cells continued in a direct relationship with time up to 60 min. At low concentrations of mannitol and short reaction times, histamine release, although small, was largely energy-dependent (Table 5.1) but with increasing mannitol concentration and longer reaction times, this energy

Table 5.1. The inhibition of mannitol-induced histamine release from two dispersed lung cell preparations by the metabolic inhibitors 2-deoxyglucose (5 mmol/litre) and anti-mycin A (1 μmol/litre) in glucose-free buffer. The net percentage histamine release and the percentage inhibition in the presence of the metabolic blockers are given both for concentrations of mannitol ranging from 0.5 to 1.0 M and for reaction times varying from 20 to 60 min. Approx 2×10^6 cells were challenged in a final volume of 200 μl

	Mannitol conc.	DL12 Time (min)			DL13 Time (min)		
		20	40	60	20	40	60
Net % release	1.0	4.5	9.8	11.6	12.3	19.6	32.8
	0.75	3.4	6.0	6.3	5.5	9.5	13.3
	0.5	4.9	7.8	6.7	5.7	4.8	5.2
% inhibition	1.0	37.8	21.4	1.7	30.9	7.1	20.4
	0.75	41.2	6.7	−19.0	54.5	34.7	31.6
	0.5	93.9	69.2	43.3	94.7	19.1	−1.9

dependency was lost. With mannitol concentrations of 0.75 M and 1.0 M, histamine release at 40 min was almost entirely lytic.

The kinetics of mannitol-induced histamine release from human bronchoalveolar cells would also be consistent with two processes. After a rapid initial increase, histamine release reaches a plateau between 5 and 20 min, and then rises more slowly to 60 min (Fig. 5.2). Once again at low concentrations of mannitol, histamine release is largely energy-dependent (Fig. 5.3).

Thus the evidence would suggest that there are two processes in the mannitol-induced release of histamine from both dispersed lung mast cells and bronchoalveolar mast cells—an initial energy-dependent process which is largely complete within 5 min and a sustained lytic process which becomes dominant after longer time intervals. This latter phase appears to be similar in both preparations as net histamine release from dispersed lung cells and bronchoal-

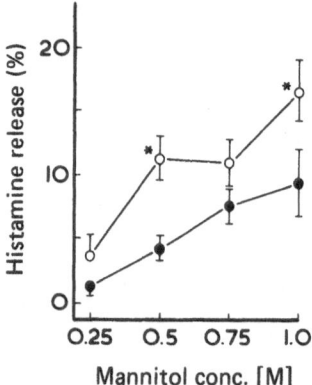

Fig. 5.3. Mannitol-induced histamine release from human bronchoalveolar cells (10 min reaction time) in full Tyrodes buffer (○) or in glucose-free Tyrodes buffer plus 2-deoxyglucose (5 mM) and anti-mycin A (1 μM) (●). The *points* represent the mean of seven experiments + SEM.

veolar cells between 20 and 60 min was similar (7.9% and 7.1% of total histamine respectively). The major difference between these two preparations lies in the early, non-lytic phase. This initial phase resulted in a net histamine release from human bronchoalveolar cells of 16.7%±3.0% (mean ± [SE], 0.75 M mannitol, 20 min) but only 4.2%±1.0% histamine release from human dispersed lung cells (0.75 M mannitol, 20 min). A similar difference in net histamine release between these two preparations is seen at 10 min.

Increased Extracellular Osmolarity and Histamine Release

Although mannitol has been proposed as a model for hyperosmolar challenge of basophils (Findlay et al. 1981) and lung mast cells (Eggleston et al. 1984), a more appropriate method of increasing extracellular osmolarity is to use increasing concentrations of solutes in physiological buffer. For this reason, further experiments were performed using as the challenge solution Tyrodes buffer containing increasing solute concentrations, such that the final concentration of all solutes ranged from two to five times the standard concentration (540–1350 mosm/kg). Manipulating extracellular osmolarity in such a way resulted in dose-dependent histamine release from bronchoalveolar cells that was similar to mannitol-induced release (Fig. 5.4) except that the plateau was more pronounced with no increase in histamine release despite increasing osmolarity from 810–1340 mosm/kg. At osmolarities of about 1000 mosm/kg or below histamine release in response to increasing solute concentrations was similar to that in

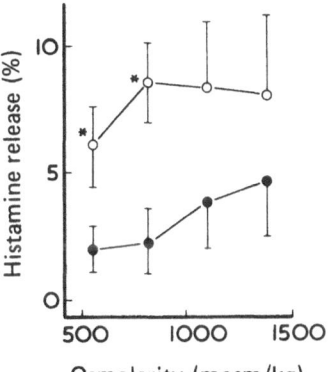

Fig. 5.4. The inhibition of histamine release from human bronchoalveolar cells in response to increasing buffer solute concentration (2–5×Tyrodes) by the metabolic inhibitors 2-deoxyglucose (5 mM) and anti-mycin A (1 μM) in glucose-free buffer. *Points* represent the mean of five paired experiments with SE bars. (○=full Tyrodes, ●=glucose-free Tyrodes with inhibitors.)

response to mannitol. The lytic effect is more pronounced at higher osmolarities and it is likely that this lytic effect will be greater with mannitol, as it will be totally excluded from the cell. Many buffer solutes will penetrate into the cell resulting in a smaller osmotic difference across the membrane. This may explain the higher levels of histamine release seen at higher osmolarities when induced by mannitol compared with increased buffer solute concentrations. Alternatively it is possible that high concentrations of extracellular ions such as calcium present in the concentrated buffer may inhibit histamine release.

Histamine release in response to hyperosmolar stimulus by increasing extracellular solute concentrations is more sensitive to depletion of metabolic energy particularly at low levels of osmotic challenge. Challenge with solutes at three times the usual concentration (810 mosm/kg) was 78% inhibited in the presence of antimycin A (1 μM) and 2-deoxyglucose (5 mM) in glucose-free medium (Fig. 5.4). As depletion of metabolic energy leads to enhancement of lytic processes because of inhibition of cellular repair, this suggests that release by hyperosmolar buffer at this level of stimulus is largely energy-dependent.

The resting osmolarity of human tracheal secretions averages 359±56 mosm/kg (Potter et al. 1967). Canine and human bronchial secretions are similarly hypertonic with respect to plasma (Mann et al. 1979; Boucher et al. 1981). There

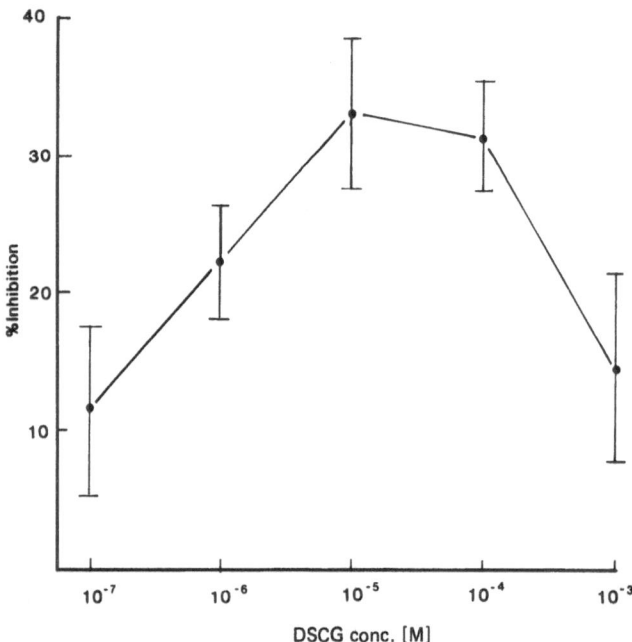

Fig. 5.5. Inhibition of mannitol-induced histamine release by disodium cromoglycate. Disodium cromoglycate was preincubated with the cells for 10 min prior to activation with 0.75 M mannitol and the reaction stopped after a further 10 min. *Points* represent the mean of six experiments with SE bars. Control release was 18.5±3.3 (SE%).

are no direct measures of the osmolarity of airway secretions during hyperventilation but estimates of water flux suggest that osmolarity will increase. Net losses of 300 ml/day from the lungs have been measured during normal tidal breathing (Cole et al. 1983) and increase with increasing levels of ventilation. At modest levels of hyperventilation (20 liter/min, inspired air 24°C, 40% relative humidity) losses reach 45 ml/h (Caldwell et al. 1969). Levels of ventilation considerably higher are required to induce post-exertional bronchoconstriction (of the order of 70 litre/ min, inspired air 25°C, 0% relative humidity: Strauss et al. 1978; Deal et al. 1979a). At this level of ventilation water losses from the respiratory tract would exceed 100 ml/h. It is likely that such losses would lead to a transient rise in the osmolarity of lung secretions to levels that could result in the release of mediators from lung mast cells.

It has been proposed that hyperosmolar histamine release from human dispersed lung mast cells might be relevant to the pathogenesis of exercise-induced asthma (Eggleston et al. 1984). Histamine release from dispersed human lung mast cells is a slow process, taking 40–60 min to achieve significant levels and at this time interval, histamine release appears to be largely lytic. Bronchoalveolar mast cells in contrast will release significant quantities of histamine within 1 min of hyperosmolar challenge. Significant and energy-dependent histamine release occurs at mannitol concentrations of 0.25 M (560 mosm/kg) and with twice concentrated Tyrodes buffer (540 mosm/kg) (mean 5.4 and 6.2% release respectively), which are close to the range of osmolarities that could be achieved in vivo. Even such low levels of histamine release in vivo are likely to have major effects on human airways. Guinea pig airway achieves 50% of its maximum contractile response in vitro to antigen at 1% net histamine release (Adams and Lichtenstein 1979).

Hyperosmolar histamine release from bronchoalveolar mast cells is inhibited by disodium cromoglycate. Even with optimal stimulation (0.75 M mannitol, 1020 mosm/kg) well beyond what is likely to be achieved in vivo, DSCG (10 M) caused 39% inhibition of histamine release (Fig. 5.5). This chromone is an effective prophylactic against exercise-induced asthma (Davies 1968) and will inhibit the bronchoconstrictor response to cold dry air (Fanta et al. 1981). Attenuation of exercise-induced asthma by DSCG is associated with inhibition of the appearance of histamine and neutrophil chemotactic factor in the peripheral blood which is compatible with inhibition of mast cell mediator release.

The speed with which bronchoalveolar mast cells respond to changes in osmolarity with an energy-dependent histamine release, suggests that these cells may play a role in the initiation of exercise-induced asthma. Lying superficially they would be exposed to hyperosmolar lung secretions and that osmolarity of such secretions is likely to increase considerably during exercise. Hyperosmolar histamine release also provides a further example of the differences between human bronchoalveolar and human dispersed lung mast cells.

References

Adams GK, Lichtenstein LM (1979) In vitro studies of antigen-induced bronchospasm: effect of anti-histamines and SRS-A antagonists on the response of sensitised guinea pig and human airways to antigen. J Immunol 122: 555–562

Anderson SD, Schoeffel RE, Daviskas E, Black JL (1983) Exercise-induced asthma without airways cooling. Am Rev Resp Dis 127: 228 (Abstr)

Barr-Orr O, Neuman I, Dotan R (1977) Effects of dry and humid climates on exercise-induced asthma in adolescents and children. J Allergy Clin Immunol 60: 163–178

Bar-Yishay E, Gur I, Inbar O, Newman I, Dlin RA, Godfrey S (1982) Difference between swimming and running as stimuli for exercise-induced asthma. Eur J Appl Physiol 48: 387–397

Bar-Yishay E, Ben-Dov I, Godfrey S (1983) Influence of airway temperature on the refractory period following hyperventilation-induced asthma. Am Rev Resp Dis 127: 572–574

Boucher RC, Stutts MJ, Bromberg PA, Gatzy JT (1981) Regional differences in airway surface liquid composition. J Appl Physiol 50: 613–620

Caldwell PRB, Gomez DM, Fritts HW (1969) Respiratory heat exchange in normal subjects and in patients with pulmonary disease. J Appl Physiol 26: 82–88

Chen WY, Horton DJ (1977) Heat and water loss from the airways and exercise-induced asthma. Respiration 34: 305–313

Cole P, Forsyth R, Haight JS (1983) The effect of cold air and exercise on nasal patency. Ann Otol Rhinol Laryngol 92: 196–198

Davies SE (1968) The effect of disodium cromoglycate on exercise-induced asthma. Br Med J 3: 593–594

Deal EC, McFadden ER, Ingram RH, Jaeger JJ (1979a) Hyperpnoea and heat flux, the initial reaction sequence in exercise-induced asthma. J Appl Physiol 46: 476–483

Deal EC, McFadden ER, Ingram RH, Jaeger JJ (1979b) Oesophageal temperature during exercise in asthmatic and non-asthmatic subjects. J Appl Physiol 46: 484–490

Deal EC, McFadden ER, Ingram RH, Strauss RH, Jaeger JJ (1979c) Role of respiratory heat exchange in the production of exercise-induced asthma. J Appl Physiol 46: 467–475

Deal EC, Wasserman SI, Soter NA, Ingram RH, McFadden ER (1980) Evaluation of role played by mediators of immediate hypersensitivity in exercise-induced asthma. J Clin Invest 65: 659–665

Edmunds AT, Tooley M, Godfrey S (1978) The refractory period after exercise-induced asthma, its duration and relation to severity of exercise. Am Rev Resp Dis 117: 247–254

Eggleston PA, Kagey-Sabotka A, Schleimer RP, Lichtenstein LM (1984) Interaction between hyperosmolar and IgE mediated histamine release from basophils and mast cells. Am Rev Resp Dis 130: 86–91

Fanta CH, McFadden ER, Ingram RH (1981) Effects of cromolyn sodium on the response to respiratory heat loss in normal subjects. Am Rev Resp Dis 123: 161–164

Findlay SR, Dvorak AM, Kagey-Sabotka A, Lichtenstein LM (1981) Hyperosmolar triggering of histamine release from human basophils. J Clin Invest 67: 1640–1643

Floyer J (1698) A treatise of the asthma. R Wilkin, London. Quoted by Sakula A. Sir John Floyer's A treatise of the asthma. Thorax 1984; 39: 248–254

Godfrey S, Silverman M, Anderson S (1973) Problems of interpreting exercise-induced asthma. J Allergy Clin Immunol 52: 199–209

Herxheimer H (1946) Hyperventilation in asthma. Lancet I: 83–87

Hook WA, Siraganian RP (1981) Influence of anions, cations and osmolarity on IgE mediated histamine release from human basophils. Immunology 43: 723–731

Lee TH, Nagy L, Nagakura T, Walport MJ, Kay AB (1982) Identification and partial characterisation of an exercise-induced neutrophil chemotactic factor in bronchial asthma. J Clin Invest 69: 889–99

Mann SFP, Adams GKIII, Proctor DF (1979) Effects of temperature, relative humidity and mode of breathing on canine airway secretions. J Appl Physiol 46: 205–210

McFadden ER, Denison DM, Waller JF, Assourfi B, Peacock A, Sopwith T (1982) Direct recordings of the temperature of the tracheobronchial tree in normal man. J Clin Invest 69: 700–705

McFadden ER, Pichurko B, Bowman KF et al. (1983) Thermal mapping of the airways in man. Fed Proc 41: 1357 (Abstr)

McFadden ER, Pichurko BM, Soter NA, Ringel EW, Melford IM (1984) Respiratory heat exchange and the asthmatic response. In: Kay AB, Austen KF, Lichtenstein LM (eds) Asthma. Physiology, immunopharmacology and treatment. Academic Press, London, pp 315–324

Nagakura T, Lee TH, Assoufi BK, Newman-Taylor AJ, Denison DM, Kay AB (1983) Neutrophil chemotactic factor in exercise and hyperventilation-induced asthma. Am Rev Resp Dis 128: 294–296

Potter JL, Matthews LW, Spector S, Lemm J (1967) Studies on pulmonary secretions II. Osmolarity and ionic environment of pulmonary secretions from patients with cystic fibrosis, bronchiectasis and laryngectomy. Am Rev Resp Dis 96: 83–89

Schleimer RP, Gillespie I, Daiuta R, Lichtenstein LM (1981) Release of histamine from human leucocytes stimulated with the tumour promoting phorbol diesters II. Interaction with other stimuli. J Immunol 226: 136–140

Schoeffel RE, Anderson S, Altounyan REC (1981) Bronchial reactivity to inhalation of ultrasonically nebulised solutions of distilled water and saline. Br Med J 283: 1285–1287

Silverman M, Anderson SD (1972) Standardisation of exercise tests in asthmatic children. J Allergy Clin Immunol 52: 882–889

Smith CM, Anderson SD (1986) Hyperosmolarity as the stimulus to asthma induced by hyperventilation? J Allergy Clin Immunol 77: 729–736

Smith RJ, Iden SS (1979) Phorbol myristate acetate induced release of granule enzymes from human neutrophils: inhibition by the calcium antagonist 8-(N,N-diethylamine)-acetyl-3,4,5-dimethyl benzoate hydrochloride. Biochem Biophys Res Commun 91: 263–271

Stearns DR, McFadden ER, Breslin FJ, Ingram JR (1981) Reanalysis of the refractory period after exercise induced-asthma. J Appl Physiol 50: 503–508

Strauss RH, McFadden ER, Ingram RH, Jaeger JJ (1977) Enhancement of exercise-induced asthma by cold air. N Engl J Med 297: 743–747

Strauss RH, McFadden ER, Ingram RH, Deal EC, Jaeger JJ (1978) Influence of heat and humidity on the airway obstruction due to exercise in asthma. J Clin Invest 61: 433–440

Weiller-Ravell D, Godfrey S (1981) Do exercise and antigen-induced asthma utilise the same pathway? J Allergy Clin Immunol 5: 391–397

Weinstein RE, Anderson JA, Kvale P, Sweet LC (1976) Effects of humidification on exercise-induced asthma. J Allergy Clin Immunol 57: 250–251

Chapter 6

Newly Generated Mediators from Human Lung Mast Cells

The major problem in identifying the structural components of slow reacting substance of anaphylaxis (SRS-A) was the small quantities in which this mediator is released (Samuelsson 1983; Parker 1982). This also applies to the identification of the component leukotrienes in experimental systems. Certain identification of leukotrienes requires reverse phase HPLC, usually after an initial extraction procedure. Leukotrienes are recognised by their characteristic ultraviolet absorption (Matthews et al. 1981; Henke et al. 1984; Morris et al. 1978; Verhagen et al. 1984) in comparison with standards run in parallel or by structural confirmation of the HPLC products by gas chromatography and mass spectrometry. Such certainty requires large quantities of the initial product and allowance must be made for losses during extraction (Morris et al. 1983). The biological assay of SRS-A activity on guinea pig ileum is more sensitive but less specific and more difficult to quantify; nevertheless, it is arguable that it is biological activity rather than structure that is important. Radioimmunoassay (RIA) provides an alternative (Aeringhaus et al. 1982). The major problem with RIA is that class specific anti-sera for the individual leukotrienes are not yet available and cross-reactivity between the leukotrienes themselves and their isomers must always be borne in mind. The quantity of product which is recognised by a particular anti-serum as LTC_4 is not necessarily the same as the quantity that would be identified by RP-HPLC followed by GC-MS.

Mediator Release from Human Dispersed Lung Mast Cells

In addition to the release of preformed granule stored mediators, IgE-dependent challenge of human lung fragments leads to the de novo synthesis of mediators from cell membrane lipids (Schulman et al. 1981). The cell type or types responsible for the major part of this synthesis have yet to be identified with certainty, but there is evidence that such newly generated mediators are of major importance in the pathogenesis of airflow obstruction in asthmatic subjects.

The generation of cyclooxygenase and lipoxygenase products of arachidonic acid metabolism by human lung mast cells has been the subject of conflicting reports. When dispersed human lung mast cells are partially purified by gradient methods, the quantities of SRS-A generated after IgE-dependent activation are reduced compared to the starting population (Lewis et al. 1981). This has led these authors to suggest that leukotriene generation following IgE-dependent mast cell activation may involve a secondary, non-mast cell type. However, dispersed human lung mast cells purified by countercurrent centrifugal elutriation and affinity chromatography retain their capacity for leukotriene generation, even in fractions purified to near homogeneity (MacGlashan et al. 1982). Although the quantity of leukotriene generated varied considerably in different experiments, there was no loss in synthetic capacity with increasing mast cell purity. An alternative hypothesis to that proposing leukotriene generation secondary to mast cell activation, but by non-mast cell species, and one which might reconcile these conflicting observations, is that there might exist in human lung a subclass of mast cell comparable to the mouse bone marrow derived mast cell and capable of generation of large quantities of leukotrienes (Lewis et al. 1984). Different methods of purification may vary in their capacity to retain this subpopulation of mast cells.

After passive sensitisation, dispersed human lung cells also show dose-dependent generation of immunoreactive PGD_2 and LTC_4 after challenge with anti-IgE. Prostaglandin D_2 generation occurs in parallel with histamine release but reaches a plateau at an anti-IgE dilution of 1/1000 and above. There is also a trend towards PGD_2 generation by dispersed lung cells at lower levels of stimulus compared with histamine, suggesting that biologically effective concentrations of this arachidonic acid metabolite may be achieved at lower levels of activation. It was found that maximal release of PGD_2 from human lung fragments required a lower antigen concentration than that required for histamine release. Similarly, using anti-IgE as the stimulus Lewis et al. (1982) state that generation of PGD_2 at dilutions of 1/ 200–1/25 were comparable and anti-IgE activation (dilutions of 1/1000–1/25) of rat mast cells resulted in PGD_2 generation which reached a plateau whilst release of the granule stored mediator β-hexosaminadase was still increasing. As a result, a direct relationship between release of β-hexaminadase and PGD_2 generation was found only for the dose-response portion of the PGD_2 release curve (Soter et al. 1983). A similar relationship between histamine release and PGD_2 generation was found here. No such plateau was found by Holgate et al. (1984) after activation of human dispersed lung cells by anti-IgE. The reason for this discrepancy is unclear but the position on the dose-response curve will depend on the affinity of the anti-IgE used. The mast cell derivation of PGD_2 is suggested by the finding of a direct correlation between its formation and the net release of histamine from dispersed lung. That PGD_2 is a mast cell product has been confirmed by studies on rat peritoneal (Soter et al. 1982) and human dispersed lung mast cells (Peters et al. 1982) purified to near homogeneity. However, in addition to disparate dose-response curves, PGD_2 generation and histamine release have been dissociated pharmacologically (Lewis et al. 1979), in response to stimulation with anti-IgE or ionophore (Peters et al. 1982; Holgate et al. 1984) and in terms of the kinetics of their IgE-dependent release shown here. Thus, although both are mast cell derived, the biochemical pathways for their generation and release are distinct.

The absolute levels of PGD_2 generated by dispersed lung mast cells in this study are somewhat higher than those previously reported. In the study of Peters et al. (1982) dispersed lung mast cells released a mean of 60.2 ng $PGD_2/10^6$ mast cells in response to challenge with an optimal dilution of anti-IgE and in that of Holgate et al. (1984) the mean PGD_2 generation was 88.7 ng/10^6 mast cells compared with 144.3 ng/10^6 mast cells in the present study. This may reflect differences in the strength of activation as histamine release in these two studies was also significantly lower (16% and 21% respectively compared with 49.66% in the present study). Lewis et al. (1982) found IgE-dependent PGD_2 generation from human dispersed lung mast cells of 39.5 ng/10^6 mast cells but the net percent histamine release is not given.

Immunoreactive leukotriene C_4 generation by passively sensitised human dispersed lung cells was dose-dependent upon anti-IgE dilution and did not plateau at low dilutions of anti-IgE, unlike PGD_2. It is likely that most if not all of this activity was leukotriene C_4 itself and not due to cross reactivity of the anti-serum with the other peptidolipid leukotrienes as LTC_4 is the major component of SRS-A produced by human dispersed lung mast cells with very little LTD_4 or LTE_4 (Peters et al. 1982). The LTC_4 dose-response curve more closely paralleled histamine release. This is demonstrated by the highly significant correlation ($r=0.8$, $P<0.001$) between the IgE-dependent release of these two mediators. In addition, after correction for the percentage of mast cells present there was a highly significant correlation between LTC_4 generation and PGD_2 generation by human dispersed lung cells ($r=0.9$, $P<0.0001$) strongly suggesting that all three mediators are mast cell derived. This is supported by the finding that human dispersed lung mast cells purified to near homogeneity release histamine and generate both PGD_2 and LTC_4 in similar quantities to unpurified preparations (MacGlashan et al. 1982; Peters et al. 1982).

Mediator Release from Human Bronchoalveolar Cells

Challenge of human bronchoalveolar lavage cells with anti-human IgE results in the dose-dependent generation of immunoreactive PGD_2 and LTC_4 in addition to histamine release (Figs. 6.1, 6.2). These two arachidonic acid metabolites have not yet been characterised further.

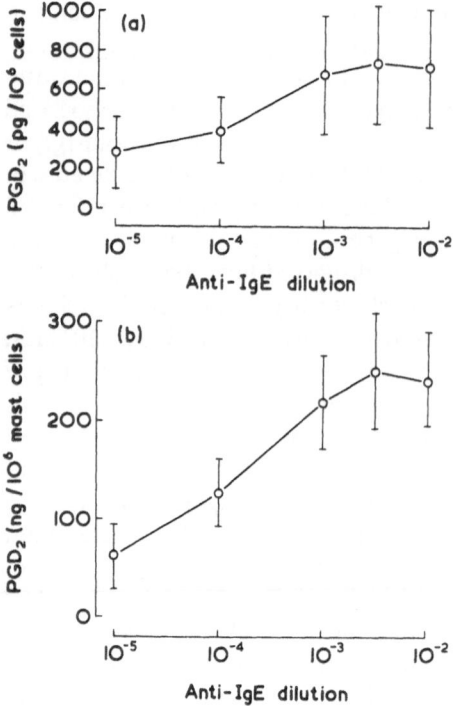

Fig. 6.1. The generation of PGD_2 by human bronchoalveolar cells in response to anti-human IgE. PGD_2 was measured by radioimmunoassay in challenged supernatants. *Points* represent the mean of 7–10 experiments with SE bars and have been corrected for spontaneous release by subtraction.

The generation of these potent inflammatory and bronchoconstrictor mediators in response to IgE-dependent challenge by cells lying superficially within the lung is likely to have profound effects in vivo. Bronchoalveolar cells recovered from a single lung subsegment are capable of releasing as much as 30 ng histamine, 16 ng of immunoreactive PGD_2 and more than 1 ng of immunoreactive LTC_4 after optimal activation via IgE-dependent mechanisms. Furthermore, mediator release occurs rapidly following activation, with significant release of the arachidonic acid metabolites within 5 min, reaching a maximum at 10 min.

The problem remains that with activation of a mixed cell population it is impossible to be certain which cell type is responsible for the major synthesis of these mediators. The correlation between net histamine release and PGD_2 generation when standardised to the mast cell number supports the hypothesis that this latter mediator is mast cell derived (Fig. 6.3). Until recently, no other

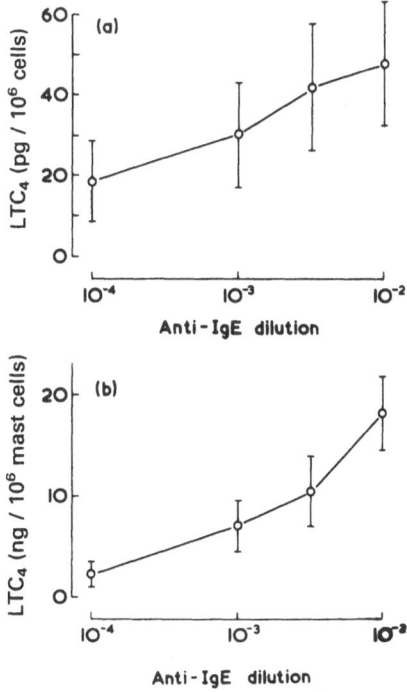

Fig. 6.2. The generation of LTC_4 by human bronchoalveolar cells in response to activation by anti-IgE. LTC_4 was measured by radioimmunoassay in challenged supernatants. *Points* represent the mean of 7–10 experiments with SE bars and have been corrected for spontaneous release by subtraction.

major cell type had been shown capable of significant PGD_2 generation but it is now clear that zymosan stimulated human alveolar macrophages will generate small quantities of PGD_2 (MacDermot et al. 1984). Similarly the cellular origin of the immunoreactive leukotriene C_4 demonstrated in supernatants after IgE-dependent challenge is unknown. In this case, no correlation could be found between the IgE-dependent release of histamine and LTC_4 generation. In part, this may be due to the highly variable background generation of this arachidonic acid metabolite. Many other cell types, including polymorphonuclear neutrophils and eosinophils and alveolar macrophages, have been shown to generate sulphidopeptide leukotrienes in response to a variety of stimuli (Aeringhaus et al. 1982). The most predominant cell in bronchoalveolar lavage is the alveolar macrophage and consequently much interest had focussed on the generation of sulphidopeptide leukotrienes by this particular cell type. The presence of IgE

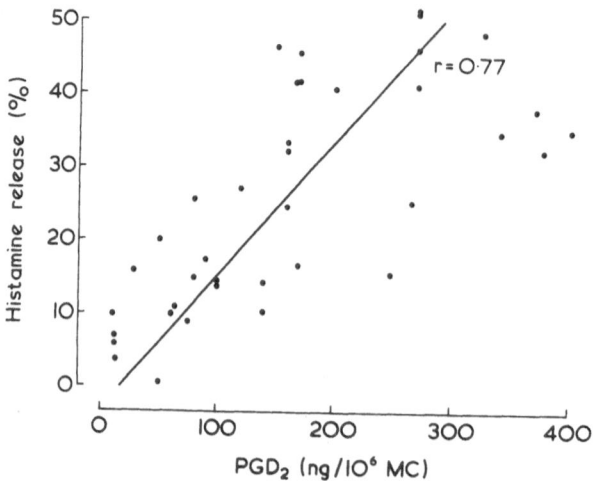

Fig. 6.3. The correlation between histamine and PGD_2 release from human bronchoalveolar cells.

receptors on cells of the monocyte-macrophage series has been amply demonstrated (Spiegelberg et al. 1983). However, the IgE-Fc receptors on macrophages are of much lower affinity than the IgE receptor of mast cells (at least 100 times) suggesting that IgE immune complexes may be more important in the activation of these cells. Leukotriene C_4 release from rat alveolar macrophages can be elicited by IgE-immune complexes (Rankin et al. 1984) but has not so far been elicited by anti-IgE. There is, however, recent evidence that anti-IgE may initiate generation of leukotriene B_4 and thromboxane B_2 from human alveolar macrophages (Fuller et al. 1985). In these circumstances anti-IgE induced release requires passive sensitisation (human myeloma IgE 10000 IU/ml) and even then generation of arachidonic acid metabolites is slow. After challenge with anti-IgE at 4°C for 30 min, thromboxane B_2 generation reached maximal levels between 15 and 45 min after increasing the temperature to 37°C. It seems unlikely therefore that primary activation of alveolar macrophages via their Fc receptors contributes significantly to the anti-IgE induced release of PGD_2 or LTC_4 measured after direct challenge of non-sensitised bronchoalveolar cells at 37°C after incubation times of only 10–15 min.

Secondary generation of arachidonic acid metabolites stimulated by primary mast cell mediator release remains a possibility. Histamine has been shown to stimulate prostanoid formation by human lung fragments (Schulman et al. 1981) and a prostaglandin generating factor of anaphylaxis (PGFA) has been described (Steel and Kaliner 1981). Released from human lung tissue after IgE-dependent stimulation, PGFA leads to the generation of PGF_2, PGE and TxB_2 from human lung tissue (Steel et al. 1982). Other cell to cell interactions, both excitatory and inhibitory are almost certain to occur and a final solution must await the purification of mast cells from bronchoalveolar lavage.

As a possible explanation for conflicting reports of leukotriene generation by partially purified human dispersed lung mast cells, it has been proposed that human lung mast cells contain a subclass comparable to the mast cells derived from mouse bone marrow in vitro (Lewis et al. 1984). Such a subclass would preferentially generate large quantities of LTC_4 and relatively less PGD_2. If such a subclass of "mucosal" type mast cells existed, it is likely that it would be predominant in bronchoalveolar lavage. Bronchoalveolar mast cells have morphological characteristics of the "mucosal" type whereas human dispersed lung contains a mixed morphological population. Nevertheless, the capacity of both preparations, human dispersed lung and bronchoalveolar mast cells, to generate PGD_2 and LTC_4 does not seem to be significantly different. If anything bronchoalveolar mast cells appear to generate marginally greater quantities of PGD_2 compared with human dispersed lung mast cells particularly as histamine release from the latter in these experiments (after passive sensitisation) was marginally better. Even assuming all of the LTC_4 detected in challenged supernatants of bronchoalveolar cells to be derived from mast cells, bronchoalveolar mast cell generation of this mediator would be comparable to human dispersed lung mast cell generation, not significantly better. There is therefore no evidence to support the hypothesis that mast cells in the bronchial mucosa of the lung generate large quantities of LTC_4 comparable to the mouse bone marrow derived mast cells. Generation of both immunoreactive LTC_4 and PGD_2 by bronchoalveolar and human dispersed lung mast cells appears to be similar, with the exception of the requirement for passive sensitisation of dispersed lung cells.

It has been demonstrated that bronchoalveolar mast cells possess distinct functional properties from dispersed human lung mast cells. Whilst it is appreciated that both preparations contain cells of different lineage, all of which may contribute to mediator synthesis, cell to cell interactions in vivo may be important in the pathogenesis of airflow obstruction, and the synthesis of mediators by the bronchoalveolar population as a whole is therefore relevant.

Newly Generated Mediators of Immediate Hypersensitivity

Unstimulated mast cells do not contain all of the mediators detected after IgE-dependent mast cell activation; some must therefore be newly generated. Because of their extraordinary biological potency, interest in recent years has focussed on such mediators synthesised de novo from membrane lipids. These mediators comprise platelet activating factor and the metabolites of arachidonic acid via two enzyme pathways: the cyclooxygenase pathway and the lipoxygenase pathway. The action of cyclooxygenase on arachidonic acid leads to the formation of prostaglandins and thromboxanes and that of 5-lipoxygenase to the formation of monohydroxy fatty acids and the leukotrienes. These mediators are not necessarily solely derived from mast cells. They are produced by a variety of cell types (Rankin et al. 1982) and their precise role in asthma has yet to be determined.

Arachidonic acid is liberated within 30 sec of membrane receptor triggering by the action of phospholipase A_2 on phosphatidyl choline. Further arachidonic acid may be produced by the action of phospholipase-C and diacyl glycerolipase. The arachidonic acid generated may then enter either of the enzyme pathways leading to the formation of either prostaglandins, thromboxanes, or leukotrienes and the monohydroxyeicosatetraenoic acids. The final products generated by any particular cell type are dependent on the presence and activation of the relevant enzymes within the cell.

Human mast cells and mast cells from other species possess the enzyme systems necessary for arachidonic acid metabolism via both the cyclooxygenase and lipoxygenase pathways. However, it is apparent that not all mast cells express these pathways to the same extent. The major cyclooxygenase product of the rat serosal mast cell is prostaglandin D_2 (Lewis et al. 1982) but chondroitin sulphate containing mast cells derived from mouse bone marrow produce little of this prostanoid after activation (Razin et al. 1982). In contrast, after IgE-dependent activation, these mouse bone marrow derived mast cells generate large quantities of LTC_4. More recently it has been demonstrated that dog mastocytoma mast cells may show similar differences in the generation of mediators of immediate hypersensitivity between cell lines. Two distinct mastocytoma cell lines passaged serially through mice differed in the lipoxygenase products generated in response to calcium ionophore. The larger cell line generated predominantly 5-hydroxy-eicosatetraenoic acid (5-HETE) and LTC_4 whereas the smaller cell line generated 12-HETE and 8,15-leukotrienes without detectable LTC_4 (Lazarus 1985). In addition, the lipoxygenase profile in response to different secretagogues differed, suggesting that the spectrum of mediators released by mast cells in response to different stimuli may also be different.

Prostaglandins and Thromboxanes

The prostaglandins were first described in seminal fluid in the 1930s and purified by Bergstrom and Sjovall (1960). The biosynthetic pathway for the production of prostaglandins and thromboxane is set out in Fig. 6.1. Prostaglandins (PG) D_2, $F_{2\alpha}$, E_2 and I_2 are formed from the endoperoxide intermediates, prostaglandins G_2 and H_2, which may also give rise to thromboxane A_2 via the action of thromboxane synthetase. The specific prostaglandin products produced by any particular cell type varies and depends upon the presence of specific enzymes capable of metabolising the endoperoxides (PGG_2 and PGH_2) to their final products. The lack of highly purified cell preparations and the short biological half life of prostaglandins makes the study of these mediators particularly difficult.

   The earliest observation of prostaglandin release after anaphylactic challenge of lung tissue was made by Piper and Vane (1969) who demonstrated a material in the venous effluent of isolated perfused guinea pig lung which on a series of smooth muscle preparations had a profile of contractile activity identical to that of prostaglandin E_2. IgE-dependent challenge of chopped human lung after passive sensitisation leads to the release of PGD_2, PGI_2, PGE_1, PGE_2, $PGF_{2\alpha}$ and thromboxane (Tx) A_2 (measured as its stable metabolite TxB_2), in variable quantities. Radioimmunoassays have shown PGD_2 and PGI_2 to be the major products with lesser quantities of the outer metabolites (Schulman et al. 1981). More recently studies of isolated human dispersed lung mast cells have demonstrated preferential generation of PGD_2 as their major cyclooxygenase product (Lewis et al. 1982) suggesting that TxA_2 and the other prostaglandins detected after activation of chopped human lung are derived from other cell types. This does not mean that they are unimportant. It is possible that cell to cell interactions within the lung after activation via IgE-dependent mechanisms leads to the production of a variety of mediators and therefore to amplification of the original response. Nevertheless, the response of individual cell types needs to be carefully identified before such interactions can be defined.

Prostaglandin D_2

Prostaglandin D_2 has been detected in supernatants after challenge of chopped human lung in vitro (Schulman et al. 1981) and is the major cyclooxygenase product of human dispersed lung mast cells (Lewis et al. 1982). This prostaglandin was originally considered to be a biologically inactive metabolite, but it has subsequently been shown to be a potent pulmonary vasoconstrictor and bronchoconstrictor in dog, monkey and man (Dawson et al. 1974; Spannhake et al. 1978; Patterson et al. 1980). It is considerably more potent than $PGF_{2\alpha}$ in its bronchoconstrictor effect in normal human subjects (Hardy et al. 1984). In addition, intradermal injection of PGD_2 in human subjects produces a wheal and flare reaction accompanied by dilatation of capillaries and venules and dermal oedema (Soter et al. 1983).

Prostaglandin $F_{2\alpha}$

In addition to $PGF_{2\alpha}$ release after challenge of chopped human lung in vitro (Schulman et al. 1981) an increase in the plasma levels of the $PGF_{2\alpha}$ metabolite (16-keto-13,14-dihydroprostaglandin $F_{2\alpha}$) has been detected after allergen provoked asthma in vivo (Green et al. 1974). This prostanoid is a potent constrictor of human bronchial smooth muscle (Sweatman and Collier 1968) and asthmatics are hyperreactive to inhaled $PGF_{2\alpha}$ in a similar way to histamine (Mathe and Hedquist 1975). Intravenous $PGF_{2\alpha}$ has less bronchoconstrictor effect, perhaps due to its different access to airway receptors (Brown et al.

1978). Alternatively, part of the bronchoconstrictor effect of $PGF_{2\alpha}$ may therefore be secondary to bronchial irritation. Inhalation of $PGF_{2\alpha}$ has been shown to stimulate lung irritant receptors (Coleridge et al. 1976) and the response to inhaled $PGF_{2\alpha}$ is partially inhibited by atropine (Mathe and Hedquist 1975).

Prostaglandin E_2

Prostaglandin E_2 intravenously or by inhalation leads to bronchodilatation in both animals and normal man (Mathe and Hedquist 1975; Walters et al. 1982). Like $PGF_{2\alpha}$, inhalation of PGE_2 is irritant, causing cough and retrosternal discomfort and perhaps because of this the response to PGE_2 inhalation in asthmatics is less predictable (Smith et al. 1975; Mathe and Hedquist 1975). Release of PGE_2-like material has been demonstrated after histamine-induced contraction of guinea pig trachea in vitro leading to the hypothesis that local PGE_2 release may be a protective bronchodilator mechanism (Grodzinska et al. 1976).

Prostacyclin (PGI_2)

Prostacyclin is most well known for its cardiovascular and platelet-active effects (Moncada 1982). It is known to relax bronchial smooth muscle in vitro (Gardiner and Collier 1980) but had little overall effect on pulmonary compliance in vivo. It may afford short-term protection against non-specific bronchoconstrictor stimuli such as exercise or water mist (Bianco et al. 1978). In one study, prostacyclin led to bronchodilation in a small subgroup of asthmatics but these could not be distinguished from the group as a whole (Hardy et al. 1985).

Slow Reacting Substances and the Leukotrienes

Slow reacting substance (SRS), defined by its ability to produce a slow sustained contraction of guinea pig ileum, was first demonstrated in perfusates of lung exposed to cobra venom (Feldberg and Kellaway 1938). A similar activity was later demonstrated after immunological challenge of guinea pig lung and called slow reacting substance of anaphylaxis (SRS-A) (Brocklehurst 1960). Because of its instability, its high affinity for proteins and its production in very small amounts, elucidation of the structure of SRS-A proved extremely difficult. Its derivation from arachidonic acid was shown by incorporation of a carbon label (Jaschik et al. 1974). Structure-elucidation began in earnest with the demonstration that SRS-A was a polar lipid with a characteristic ultraviolet absorption (Morris et al. 1978). Large quantities of SRS were produced by ionophore stimulation of mouse mastocytoma cells and purified after extraction by high pressure liquid chromatography (HPLC). The structure was then deduced by chemical and enzymic degradation (Hammerstrom et al. 1979) and finally confirmed by total chemical synthesis (Hammerstrom et al. 1980). Characterisation of an immunologically released SRS-A from guinea pig lung followed shortly afterwards (Morris et al. 1983).

The family of peptidolipids making up the activity of SRS-A have been called the leukotrienes (LT). The initial step in leukotriene production is the enzymic conversion of arachidonic acid to 5-hydroperoxyeicosatetraenoic acid (5-HPETE) in the presence of the 5-lipoxygenase enzyme. This has been identified as the initial step in the rat basophil leukaemic cells (Orning et al. 1980), neutrophils (Borgeat and Samuelsson 1979), alveolar macrophages (Fels et al. 1982) and mouse mast cells (Razin et al. 1982). 5-HPETE is then either reduced to 5-hydroxyeicostetraenoic acid (5-HETE) or enters the leukotriene pathway (Fig. 6.2). The specific 5-lipoxygenase products produced by any particular cell type depend on the presence of particular enzymes for each of the metabolic steps in a similar way to the production of the final prostaglandin products of the cyclooxygenase pathway. The initial leukotriene product (LTA$_4$) may be transformed to 5,12-dihydroxyeicosatetraenoic acid (LTB$_4$) [catalysed by soluble epoxide hydrolase] (Jaschik and Kuo 1983) or by the addition of glutathione [glutathione-s-transferase] to leukotriene C$_4$ (Jaschik et al. 1982). Non-enzymatic hydrolysis of LTA$_4$ to 6-transLTB$_4$ or 5,6-dihydroxy-eicosatetraenoic acid also occurs to a significant extent in some cell types. The removal of the terminal glutamine from LTC$_4$ by gammaglutamyl transpeptidase leads to the production of LTD$_4$ and the action of dipeptidases in plasma and tissues to LTE$_4$ (Lee et al. 1983a; Krilis et al. 1983). The sulphidopeptide leukotrienes LTC$_4$, LTD$_4$ and LTE$_4$ together constitute the biological activities of SRS-A (Morris et al. 1983; Bach et al. 1980).

SRS-A Production

The generation of SRS-A has been demonstrated after anaphylactic challenge of guinea pig lung (Brocklehurst 1960) and after IgE-dependent challenge of passively sensitised human lung fragments (Parish 1967; Sheard et al. 1967). SRS-A generation in vitro has more recently been demonstrated after antigen challenge of lung fragments from asthmatic subjects (Hannsen et al. 1983) where SRS-A release occurred in parallel with contraction of bronchial smooth muscle. There is evidence that isolated mast cells have the capacity to generate SRS-A/leukotrienes but that this is not necessarily a universal property of all mast cells. Rat serosal mast cells will elaborate SRS-A after challenge with calcium ionophore but not after IgE-dependent challenge (Yecies et al. 1979). In contrast mouse bone marrow derived mast cells elaborate large quantities of leukotrienes after activation with either ionophore or anti-IgE (Razin et al. 1982). The generation of leukotrienes by human dispersed lung mast cells has been the subject of recent debate. It now seems clear that isolated human dispersed lung mast cells purified to relative homogeneity have the capacity to elaborate leukotrienes after IgE-dependent activation (MacGlashan et al. 1982) although whether this is the property of a subclass of lung mast cells remains to be determined (see earlier).

Biological Effects

The leukotrienes possess a variety of biological actions which can be demonstrated even at very low concentration.

All three sulphidopeptide leukotrienes (LTC_4, LTD_4 and LTE_4) will contract the smooth muscle of guinea pig ileum and molar ratios for equal potency are 4:2:1.5 (Lewis et al. 1980). The conversion of LTC_4 to LTD_4 does not affect this contractile activity, but the conversion of LTD_4 to LTE_4 by mucosal dipeptidases with consequent loss of activity is responsible for the lack of sustained response to LTD_4 (Krilis et al. 1983).

Leukotrienes when inhaled or given intravenously possess the unique capacity to preferentially effect the compliance of guinea pig lung compared with conductance, an effect compatible with predominant activity on peripheral airways (Drazen et al. 1980, 1982; Weichman et al. 1982). Leukotriene C_4 and D_4 are also potent constrictors of human bronchial smooth muscle in vitro, LTC_4 being 1000 times more potent than histamine and 500 times more potent than $PGF_{2\alpha}$ on a molar basis (Dahlen et al. 1980). In vivo, in normal human subjects, LTC_4 and LTD_4 are approximately equipotent in inducing bronchoconstriction each being 100–9000 times more potent than histamine and with more sustained effect (Weiss et al. 1982, 1983; Holroyde et al. 1981). Measurement of the density dependence of airflow obstruction with helium oxygen mixtures suggests predominantly peripheral airway action similar to guinea pig lung (Weiss et al. 1982). Quantitatively similar effects have been observed in asthmatic subjects where inhalation produces prolonged bronchoconstriction of rapid onset (Griffin et al. 1983). Surprisingly these subjects did not show the hyperreactivity to LTD_4 characteristic of their response to histamine or $PGF_{2\alpha}$. Airway constriction in asthmatics resulted from inhalation of 1/100–1/300 of the concentration of histamine required in normal subjects but only one-third of the concentration of LTD_4. This would suggest that separate and predominantly peripheral receptors for leukotrienes are present in bronchial smooth muscle when compared with histamine and prostaglandins.

Leukotrienes will also increase capillary permeability leading to inflammatory oedema. As little as 1 nmol of LTC_4 or LTD_4 elicits a wheal and flare after intradermal injection in human subjects (Soter et al. 1983). The wheal is accompanied by dermal oedema and increased capillary permeability lasting from 2–4 h. In nanogram quantities they will induce secretion in human bronchial mucosal explants in vitro (Coles et al. 1983; Marom et al. 1982). Other, recently demonstrated properties include decrease in cardiac contractility and coronary blood flow (Burke et al. 1982; Woodman and Dusting 1982), systemic hypotension (Drazen et al. 1980) and suppression of lymphocyte function (Webb et al. 1982).

Metabolic pathways for the inactivation of leukotrienes in vivo are ill-defined. The local conversion of LTC_4 to LTD_4 to LTE_4 appears to modulate the contractile response of guinea pig ileal smooth muscle strips, the conversion of LTD_4 to LTE_4 by mucosal dipeptidases being responsible for considerable loss of contractile activity with time (Krilis et al. 1983). Leukotriene C_4 is rapidly transformed in the circulation to LTD_4 and LTE_4 such that 99% is converted within 15 min (Hammerstrom et al. 1981). All three may be inactivated by polymorphonuclear leucocytes in vitro by the myeloperoxidase-chloride dependent generation of hypochlorous acid (Lee et al. 1983b) but the precise contribution of these pathways to the in vivo metabolism of these mediators is unknown.

Platelet Activating Factor

Platelet activating factor (PAF) is a phospholipid mediator which was originally found to be released after IgE-dependent activation of rabbit basophils and identified by its ability to aggregate platelets from rabbits (Cazenave et al. 1979) and humans (Chignard et al. 1979). Naturally occurring PAF has now been structurally identified as 1-alkyl,2-acetyl s-glyceryl,3-phosphoryl choline (Demopolous et al. 1979). In addition to its ability to elicit platelet aggregation, PAF will cause platelet dependent bronchoconstriction (Vargaftig et al. 1980; Halonen et al. 1981) which may be secondary to the release of platelet SRS (Mencia-Huerta et al. 1983; Voekel et al. 1982). Other demonstrated activities include aggregation and stimulation of neutrophil oxidative metabolism (Goetzl et al. 1980; Camussi et al. 1981) and thromboxytopenia, neutropenia and basopenia (McManus et al. 1981).

IgE-dependent release of PAF from rabbit lung has been demonstrated (Kravis and Henson 1975), but the cell type or types responsible is uncertain. Numerous cell types are capable of PAF generation including alveolar macrophages (Arnoux et al. 1980), human neutrophils, basophils (Clark et al. 1980) and mast cells (Mencia-Huerta et al. 1983).

References

Aeringhaus U, Wobling RH, Kohnig W, Patrono C, Peskar BM, Peskar BA (1982) Release of leukotriene C_4 from human polymorphonuclear leukocytes as determined by radioimmunoassay. FEBS Lett 146: 111–115
Anderson CL, Spiegelberg HL (1981) Macrophage receptors for IgE: binding of IgE to specific Fc receptors on human macrophage cell line U937. J Immunol 126: 2470–2473

Arnoux B, Duval D, Benveniste J (1980) Release of platelet-activating factor (PAF acether) from alveolar macrophages by calcium ionophore A23187 and phagocytosis. Eur J Clin Invest 10: 437–441

Bach MK, Brashler JR, Hammerstrom S, Samuelsson B (1980) Identification of a component of rat mononuclear cell SRS as leukotriene D. Biochem Biophys Res Commun 93: 1121–1126

Barrett KE, Metcalfe DD (1984) Mast cell heterogeneity: Evidence and implications. J Clin Immunol 4: 253–261

Bergstrom S, Sjovall J (1960) The isolation of prostaglandin F from sheep prostate glands. Acta Chem Scand 14: 1693–1700

Bianco S, Robuschi M, Cesarani R, Gandolfi C, Kamburoff P (1978) Prevention of a specifically induced bronchoconstriction by PGI_2 and 20-methyl PGI_2 in asthmatic patients. Pharmacol Res Commun 10: 657–675

Borgeat P, Samuelsson B (1979) Arachidonic acid metabolism in polymorphonuclear leucocytes: effects of ionophore A23187. Proc Natl Acad Sci USA 76: 2148–2152

Brocklehurst WE (1960) The release of histamine and formation of a slow reacting substance (SRS-A) during anaphylactic shock. J Physiol (Lond) 151: 416–435

Brown MJ, Ind PW, Causon R, Lee TH (1982) A novel double isotope technique for the enzymatic assay of plasma histamine: application to estimation of mast cell activation assessed by antigen challenge in asthmatics. J Allergy Clin Immunol 69: 20–24

Brown R, Ingram RH, McFadden ER (1978) Effect of $F_{2\alpha}$ on lung mechanics in non-asthmatic and asthmatic subjects. J Appl Physiol 42: 221–227

Burke JA, Levi R, Guo ZG, Corey EJ (1982) Leukotrienes C_4, D_4 and E_4: effects on human and guinea pig cardiac preparations in vitro. J Pharmacol Exp Ther 221: 235–241

Camussi G, Tetta C, Bussolini F, Capio FC, Coda R, Masera C, Secolini G (1981) Mediators of immune complex-induced aggregation of polymorphonuclear neutrophils. II. Platelet activating factor as the effector substance of immune-induced aggregation. Int Arch Allergy Appl Immunol 64: 25–41

Cazenave JP, Benveniste J, Mustard JF (1979) Aggregation of rabbit platelets by platelet activating factor is independent of the release reaction and the arachidonate pathway and inhibited by membrane active drugs. Lab Invest 41: 275–280

Chignard M, Le Coedic JP, Tence M, Vargaftig BB, Benveniste J (1979) The role of platelet activating factor in platelet aggregation. Nature 279: 799–800

Clark PO, Hanahan DJ, Pinckard RN (1980) Physical and chemical properties of platelet-activating factor obtained from human neutrophils and monocytes and rabbit neutrophils and basophils. Biochem Biophys Acta 628: 69–75

Coleridge HM, Coleridge JCG, Ginzel KH, Baker DG, Banzett RB, Morrison MA (1976) Stimulation of irritant receptors and C fibres in the lungs by prostaglandins. Nature 264: 451–453

Coles SJ, Neil KH, Reid LM, Austen KF, Nii Y, Corey EJ, Lewis RA (1983) Effects of leukotriene C_4 and D_4 on glycoprotein and lysosyme section by human bronchial mucosa. Prostaglandins 25: 155–170

Dahlen SE, Hedquist P, Hammerstrom S, Samuelsson D (1980) Leukotrienes are potent bronchoconstrictors of bronchial smooth muscle. Nature 288: 484–486

Dawson W, Lewis RL, McMahon RE, Sweatman WJF (1974) Potent bronchoconstrictor activity of 15-keto prostaglandin F_2. Nature 250: 331–332

Demopolous CA, Pinckard RN, Hanahan DJ (1979) Platelet activating factor. Evidence for 1-O-alkyl-2-acetyl-sn-glyceryl-3-phosphoryl choline as the active component (a new class of lipid chemical mediators). J Biol Chem 294: 9355–9358

Drazen JM, Austen KF, Lewis RA et al. (1980) Comparative airway and vascular effects of leukotriene C and D in vivo and in vitro. Proc Natl Acad Sci USA 77: 4354–4358

Drazen JM, Venugopalan CS, Austen KF, Brion F, Corey EJ (1982) Effects of LTE on pulmonary mechanics in the guinea pig. Am Rev Resp Dis 125: 290–294

Feldberg W, Kellaway CH (1938) The liberation of histamine and the formation of lysolecithin-like substances by cobra venom. J Physiol (Lond) 94: 187–226

Fels AOS, Pawlowski NA, Cramer EB, King TKC, Cohn ZA, Scott WA (1982) Human alveolar macrophages produce leukotriene B_4. Proc Natl Acad Sci USA 76: 7866–7870

Fuller RW, Kemeny DM, Holgate ST, Morris PK, Dollery CT, MacDermott J (1985) Mediators released from human alveolar macrophages by IgE/anti-IgE complexes. Thorax 40: 716p

Gardiner PJ, Collier HO (1980) Specific receptors for prostaglandins in airways. Prostaglandins 19: 819–841

Goetzl EJ, Derian KK, Tauber AI, Valone FH (1980) Novel effects of 1-O-hexadecyl-2-acyl-sn-glycero-3-phosphoryl choline mediators on human leucocyte function: delineation of the specific role of the acyl substituents. Biochem Biophys Res Commun 94: 881–888

Green K, Hedquist P, Svanborn N (1974) Increased plasma levels of 15-keto-13,14-dihydro-prostaglandin F_2 after allergen provoked asthma in man. Lancet II: 1419–1421

Griffin MO, Weiss JW, Leitch AG, McFadden ER, Corey EJ, Austen KF, Drazen JM (1983) Airway effects of leukotriene D in asthma. N Engl J Med 308: 436–439

Grodzinska L, Pacenko B, Grydewski R (1976) Inhibition of release of prostaglandin E-like material by non-steroid and steroid anti-inflammatory drugs. Acta Biol Med Ger 35: 1099–1100

Halonen M, Palmer JD, Lohman IG, McManus LM, Pinckard RN (1981) Differential effects of platelet depletion on the physiologic alterations of IgE anaphylaxis and acetyl glyceryl ether phosphoryl choline infusion in the rabbit. Am Rev Resp Dis 124: 416–421

Hammerstrom S, Bernstrom K, Orning L, Dahlen SE, Hedquist P (1981) Rapid in vivo metabolism of leukotriene C_3 in the monkey *Macaca iris*. Biochem Biophys Res Commun 101: 1109–1115

Hammerstrom S, Murphy RC, Samuelsson B, Clark DA, Mioskowski C, Corey EJ (1979) Structure of leukotriene C. Identification of the aminoacid part. Biochem Biophys Res Commun 91: 1266–1272

Hammerstrom S, Samuelsson B, Clark DA, Goto G, Marfat A, Mioskowski C, Corey EJ (1980) Stereochemistry of leukotriene C_1. Biochem Biophys Res Commun 92: 946–953

Hannsen G, Bjork T, Dahlen SE, Hedquist P, Granstrom E, Dahlen B (1983) Specific allergen induces contraction of bronchi and formation of leukotriene C_4, D_4 and E_4 in human asthmatic lung. Adv LT PG TX Res 12: 153–157

Hardy CC, Robinson C, Tattersfield AE, Holgate ST (1984) The bronchoconstrictor effect of inhaled prostaglandin D_2 in normal and asthmatic men. N Engl J Med 311: 209–213

Hardy CC, Robinson C, Lewis RA, Tattersfield AE, Holgate ST (1985) Airway and cardiovascular responses to inhaled prostacyclin in normal and asthmatic subjects. Am Rev Resp Dis 131: 18–21

Henke DC, Kouzan S, Eling TE (1984) Analysis of leukotrienes, prostaglandins and other oxygenated metabolites of arachidonic acid by high performance liquid chromatography. Analytical Biochem 140: 87–94

Holgate ST, Burns GB, Robinson C, Church MK (1984) Anaphylactic and calcium-dependent generation of prostaglandin D_2, thromboxane B_2 and other cyclooxygenase products of dispersed human lung cells and relationship to histamine release. J Immunol 133: 2138–2144

Holroyde MC, Altounyan REC, Cole M, Dixon M, Elliott EV (1981) Bronchoconstriction produced in man by leukotrienes C and D. Lancet II: 17–18

Jaschick BA, Kuo CG (1983) Characterisation of leukotriene A_4 and B_4 synthesis. Prostaglandins 25: 762–782

Jaschick BA, Falkenheim S, Parker CW (1974) The precursor role of arachidonic acid in release of slow reacting substance from rat basophilic leukaemic cells. Proc Natl Acad Sci USA 74: 4577–4581

Jaschick BA, Harper T, Murphy RC (1982) Leukotriene C_4 and D_4 formation by particulate enzymes. J Biol Chem 257: 5346–5349

Kravis TC, Henson PM (1975) IgE-induced release of a platelet activating factor from rabbit lung. J Immunol 115: 1677–1681

Krilis S, Lewis RA, Corey EJ, Austen KF (1983) Bioconversion of C_6 sulphidopeptide leukotrienes by the responding guinea pig ilium determines the time course of its contraction. J Clin Invest 71: 909–915

Lazarus SC (1985) Mast cell derived mediators and their role in cell to cell interactions in the airways. International Symposium on Reversible Airways Obstruction. Neurohumoral Mechanisms and Treatment. Florence. Pergamon, Oxford, p 13

Lee CW, Lewis RA, Corey EJ, Austen KF (1983a) Conversion of leukotriene D_4 to leukotriene E_4 by a dipeptidase released from the specific granule of human polymorphonuclear leucocytes. Immunology 48: 27–35

Lee CW, Lewis RA, Tauber AI, Mehrotra MM, Corey EJ, Austen KF (1983b) The myeloperoxidase-dependent metabolism of leukotriene C_4, D_4 and E_4 to 6 trans-leukotriene B_4 diastereoisomers and the subclass specific s-diastereoisomeric sulfoxides. J Biol Chem 258: 15004–15010

Lewis RA, Holgate ST, Roberts JLII, Maguire JF, Oates JA, Austen KF (1979) Effects of indomethacin on cyclic nucleotide levels and histamine release from rat serosal mast cells. J Immunol 123: 1663–1668

Lewis RA, Drazen JM, Austen KF, Clark DA, Corey EJ (1980) Identification of the C(6)-s-conjugate of leukotriene A with cysteinic as a naturally occurring slow reacting substance of anaphylaxis (SRS-A). Importance of the 11-cis geometry for biological activity. Biochem Biophysiol Res Commun 96: 271–277

Lewis RA, Drazen JM, Corey EJ, Austen KF (1981) Structural and functional characteristics of the leukotriene components of slow reacting substance of anaphylaxis (SRS-A). In: Piper PJ (ed) SRS-A and the leukotrienes. Wiley, London pp 101–117

Lewis RA, Soter NA, Diamond PT, Austen KF, Oates JA, Roberts LJ (1982) Prostaglandin D_2 generation after activation of rat and human mast cells with anti-IgE. J Immunol 129: 1627–1631

Lewis RA, Mencia-Huerta JM, Lee CW, Austen KF (1984) Mast cell dependent synthesis of lipid mediators of immediate hypersensitivity. In: Kay AB, Austen KF, Lichtenstein LM (eds) Asthma physiology, immunopharmacology and treatment. Academic Press, London pp 63–83

MacDermot J, Kelsey CR, Waddell KA, Richmond R, Knight RK, Cole PJ, Dollery CT, Landon DN, Blair IA (1984) Synthesis of leukotriene B_4 and prostanoids by human alveolar macrophages: analysis by gas chromatography and mass spectrometry. Prostaglandins 27: 163–179

MacGlashan DW, Schleimer RP, Peters SP et al. (1982) Generation of leukotrienes by purified human lung mast cells. J Clin Invest 70: 747–751

Marom Z, Shelhamer JH, Bach MK, Morton DR, Kaliner M (1982) Slow reacting substances leukotrienes C_4 and D_4 increase the release of mucus from human airways in vitro. Am Rev Resp Dis 126: 449–451

Mathe AA, Hedquist D (1975) Effects of PGF_2 and E_2 on airway conductance in healthy subjects and asthmatic patients. Am Rev Resp Dis 111: 313–320

Matthews WR, Rokach J, Murphy RC (1981) Analysis of leukotrienes by high pressure liquid chromatography. Analytical Biochem 118: 96–101

McManus LM, Pinckard RN, Fitzpatrick FA, O'Rourke RA, Crawford MH, Hanahan DJ (1981) Acetyl glyceryl ether phosphoryl choline: intravascular alterations following intravenous infusions in the baboon. Lab Invest 45: 303–307

Mencia-Huerta JM, Lewis RA, Razin E, Austen KF (1983) Antigen initiated release of platelet activating factor (PAF acether) from mouse bonemarrow derived mast cells sensitised with monoclonal IgE. J Immunol 131: 2958–2964

Moncada S (1982) Biological importance of prostacyclin. Br J Pharmacol 76: 3–31

Morris HR, Taylor GW, Piper PJ, Sirois P, Tippins JR (1978) Slow reacting substance of anaphylaxis: purification and characterisation. FEBS Lett 87: 203–206

Morris HR, Taylor GW, Piper PJ, Tippins JR (1983) The structure of slow reacting substance of anaphylaxis from guinea pig lung. Nature 285: 104–105

Morris HR, Taylor GW, Clinton PM et al. (1983) Measurement of leukotriene in asthmatics. Adv Prostaglandin Thromboxane Leukotriene Res ii: 221–223

Orning L, Hammerstrom S, Samuelsson B (1980) Leukotriene D: a slow reacting substance from rat basophil leukaemic cells. Proc Natl Acad Sci USA 77: 2014–2017

Parish WE (1967) Release of histamine and slow reacting substance with mast cell changes after challenge of human lung sensitised with reagin in vitro. Nature 215: 738–739

Parker CW (1982) Leukotrienes: their metabolism, structure and role in allergic disease. Adv Prostaglandin Thromboxane Leukotriene Res 9: 115–128

Patterson R, Harris KE, Greenberger PA (1980) Effects of prostaglandin D_2 and I_2 on the airways of rhesus monkeys. J Allergy Clin Immunol 65: 269–273

Peters SP, Schulman ES, Schleimer RP, MacGlashan DW, Newball HH, Lichtenstein LM (1982) Dispersed human lung mast cells. Pharmacologic aspects and comparison with human lung tissue fragments. Am Rev Resp Dis 126: 1034–1039

Piper PJ, Vane JR (1969) Release of additional factors in anaphylaxis and its antagonism by anti-inflammatory drugs. Nature 223: 29–35

Rankin JA, Hitchcock M, Merrill WW, Bach MK, Brashler JR, Askenase PW (1982) IgE-dependent release of leukotriene C_4 from alveolar macrophages. Nature 297: 329–331

Rankin JA, Hitchcock M, Merrill WW et al. (1984) IgE immune complexes induce immediate and prolonged release of leukotriene C_4 from rat alveolar macrophages. J Immunol 132: 1993–1999

Razin E, Mencia-Huerta JM, Lewis RA, Corey EJ, Austen KF (1982) Generation of leukotriene C_4 from a subclass of mast cells differentiated in vitro from mouse bone marrow. Proc Natl Acad Sci USA 79: 4665–4667

Samuelsson B (1983) Leukotrienes: A new class of lipid mediators of immediate hypersensitivity reactions and inflammation. Adv Prostaglandin Thromboxane Leukotriene Res 11: 1–15

Schulman ES, Newball HH, Demers LM, Fitzpatrick FA, Adkinson NF (1981) Anaphylactic release of thromboxane A_2, prostaglandin D_2 and prostacyclin from human lung parenchyma. Am Rev Resp Dis 124: 402–406

Sheard P, Killingback PG, Blair AMJ (1967) Antigen-induced release of histamine and SRS from human lung passively sensitised with reaginic serum. Nature. 216: 283–284

Smith AP, Cuthbert MF, Dunlop LS (1975) Effects of inhaled prostaglandin E_1, E_2 and F_2 on the airways of healthy and asthmatic man. Clin Sci Mol Med 48: 421–430

Soter NA, Lewis RA, Corey EJ, Austen KF (1983) Local effects of synthetic leukotrienes in human skin. J Invest Dermatol 80: 115–119

Spannhake EW, Lemen RJ, Wegman MJ, Hyman AL, Kadowicz PJ (1978) Effects of arachidonic acid and prostaglandins on lung function in the intact dog. J Appl Physiol 44: 397–405

Spiegelberg HL, Boltz-Nitulescu G, Plummer JM, Melewicz F (1983) Characterisation of IgE Fc receptors on monocytes and macrophages. Fed Proc 42: 124–128

Steel LK, Bach D, Kaliner MA (1982) Prostaglandin generating factor of anaphylaxis. II Characteristics of activity. J Immunol 129: 1233–1237

Steel LK, Kaliner MA (1981) Prostaglandin generating factor of anaphylaxis: identification and isolation. J Biol Chem 256: 12692–12698

Sweatman JF, Collier HO (1968) Effect of prostaglandin on human bronchial smooth muscle. Nature 217: 69

Vargaftig BB, Lefort J, Chignard M, Benveniste J (1980) Platelet activating factor induces a platelet dependent bronchoconstriction unrelated to the formation of prostaglandin derivatives. Eur J Pharmacol 65: 185–192

Verhagen J, Walstra P, Veldink GA, Vliegenhart JFG (1984) Separation and quantitation of leukotrienes by reversed phase high performance liquid chromatography. Prostaglandins Leukotrienes Med 13: 15–20

Voekel NF, Worthen S, Reeves JT, Henson PM, Murphy RC (1982) Non-immunological production of leukotrienes induced by platelet activating factor. Science 218: 286–288

Walters EH, Bevan A, Davies BH (1982) Interactions between the response to inhaled PGE_2 and beta-adrenergic agonist treatment. Thorax 37: 430–433

Webb DR, Nowowieski I, Healy C, Rogers TJ (1982) Immunosuppressive properties of leukotriene D_4 and E_4 in vitro. Biochem Biophys Res Commun 104: 1617–1622

Weichman BM, Muccitelli R, Osborn RR, Holden DA, Gleason JG, Wasserman MA (1982). In vitro and in vivo mechanisms of leukotriene mediated bronchoconstriction in the guinea pig. J Pharmacol Exp Ther 222: 202–208

Weiss JW, Drazen JM, Coles N, McFadden ER, Weller PF, Corey EJ, Lewis RA, Austen KF (1982) Bronchoconstrictor effects of leukotriene C in humans. Science 216: 196–198

Weiss JW, Drazen JM, McFadden ER, Weller PF, Corey EJ, Lewis RA, Austen KF (1983) Airway constriction in normal volunteers by inhalation of leukotriene D. J Am Med Ass 249: 2814–2820

Woodman OC, Dusting GJ (1982) Coronary vasoconstriction induced by leukotrienes in the anaesthetized dog. Eur J Pharmacol 86: 125–128

Yecies LD, Wedner HJ, Johnson M, Jaschick BA, Parker CW (1979) Slow reacting substance (SRS) from ionophore stimulated peritoneal mast cells of the normal rat. I. Conditions of generation and initial characterisation. J Immunol 122: 2083–2089

Chapter 7

Bronchoalveolar Mast Cells and Asthma

The preceding chapters have demonstrated that bronchoalveolar lavage provides a useful model for the study of human mast cell function. Briefly, bronchoalveolar mast cells respond to IgE-dependent challenge with histamine release and in association with other cells in the bronchoalveolar population are capable of IgE-dependent generation of leukotriene C_4 and prostaglandin D_2. In addition, mediator release can be inhibited by a variety of anti-allergic compounds. One of the major advantages of the bronchoalveolar mast cell preparation over human dispersed lung mast cells is that bronchoalveolar cells can be recovered by lavage of subjects with diverse underlying diseases allowing the study in vitro of the function of mast cells from different pathological conditions.

In view of the superficial position of mast cells, the condition in which bronchoalveolar mast cell function is of most potential interest is asthma. The mucosal surface of the lung is the first site of contact with inhaled allergens. The response of mast cells in close association with this mucosal surface may therefore be of fundamental importance to our understanding of the pathogenesis of this disease. Much of the evidence for the involvement of mast cells in human asthma remains indirect. The recovery of cells from the mucosal surface of the lung of asthmatic subjects will allow the direct demonstration of the properties of mast cells most readily accessible to antigen.

In the subjects studied, with asthma ranging from mild to moderate severity, bronchoalveolar lavage (BAL) was performed without serious adverse effects (Flint et al. 1985). This is in agreement with several other reports on the safety of BAL in asthmatic subjects (Goddard et al. 1982; Joseph et al. 1983; Diaz et al. 1984) and with the findings of the recent National Heart, Lung and Blood Institute workshop on the investigative use of BAL in asthmatics (NHLBI Workshop 1985). With the use of prewarmed isotonic solutions throughout the procedure in this study, endoscopically visible bronchoconstriction was confined to the segment lavaged. The fall in FEV_1, at the time of the procedure (mean 27%) was largely corrected by nebulised salbutamol (5 mg), and all of the subjects undergoing BAL were able to be discharged the following day.

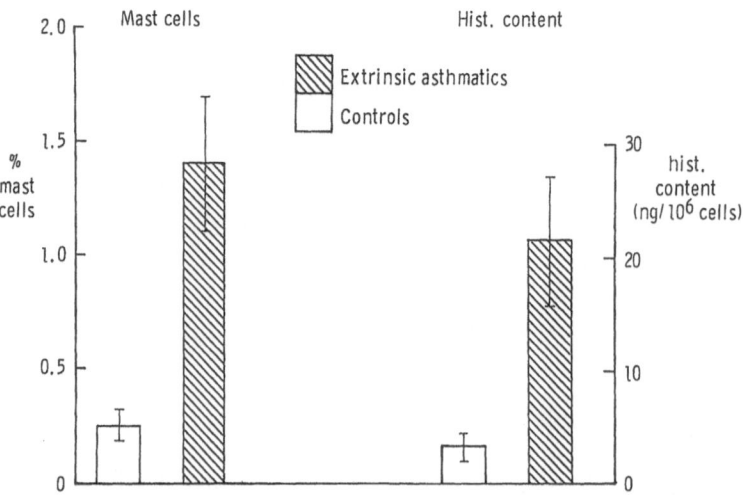

Fig. 7.1. Histogram showing difference between control subjects and patients with extrinsic asthma for percent of mast cells recovered by bronchoalveolar lavage and the histamine content of these cells.

Extrinsic Asthma

In subjects with extrinsic asthma, increased numbers of mast cells were present in the bronchoalveolar cell population, with a corresponding increase in the histamine content (Fig. 7.1) (Flint et al. 1985). Surprisingly, in view of the small numbers of subjects and the inherent variability of bronchoalveolar lavage, significant inverse correlations were found between the percentage of mast cells and the spirometric indices (FEV_1 % predicted, FEV_1/FVC ratio) and the degree of hyperreactivity to histamine (measured as the Pc 20 hist.) (Table 7.1). Similar significant correlations were seen for the relationship between the histamine content of bronchoalveolar cells and the spirometric indices, but the correlation with Pc 20 hist. failed to reach significance. This association provides indirect evidence to support the hypothesis that bronchoalveolar mast cells may be involved in the pathogenesis of airflow obstruction.

An alternative explanation for the association between the recovery of mast cells by BAL and the severity of airflow obstruction could be that the distribution of lavage fluid is affected by the presence of bronchoconstriction. Thus, bronchoalveolar cells in asthmatic subjects might be recovered from different, perhaps more proximal areas of the bronchial tree resulting in the observed increase in the percentage of mast cells. Although there was a trend for less fluid and fewer cells to be recovered from subjects with more severe asthma, this explanation is less likely for several reasons. Overall, the total recovery of cells and fluid was similar in the two groups and with the exception of mast cells

Table 7.1. Correlation coefficient for comparisons between spirometric indices, Pc20 histamine, the histamine content of BAL, percentage of mast cells and spontaneous release of histamine during a 10 minute incubation

	Histamine content	Mast cells	Spontaneous release
Fev$_1$% predicted	−0.74	−0.72	−0.12
	P<0.01	P<0.01	N.S.
FEV$_1$/FVC	−0.79	−0.76	−0.26
	P<0.005	P<0.005	N.S.
Pc20 histamine	−0.46	−0.60	−0.35
	N.S.	P<0.05	N.S.
Histamine content	–	0.88	0.54
		P<0.001	P<0.1>0.05
Mast cells	0.88	–	0.39
	P<0.001		N.S.

and eosinophils, the differential cell counts were similar in controls and asthmatics of differing severity (Table 7.2). There was no increase in the percentage of neutrophils and decrease in viability that might be expected with a more proximal lavage. In addition, in early experiments in control subjects it was found that the proportion of mast cells in the first 60 ml of lavage fluid, said to represent proximal airways, was no different from the proportion in subsequent 60 ml aliquots (unpublished observations). Finally the total number of mast cells and the total quantity of histamine recovered by BAL in asthmatic subjects is greater in all but the mildest asthmatics than in controls. As a large volume (>100 ml) lavage would be expected to reach the surface of most of the subsegment lavaged, this suggests a true increase in the number of mast cells accessible to BAL within that subsegment.

Table 7.2. The percentage of instilled fluid recovered, the total cells ($\times 10^6$) and the differential cell counts in ten subjects with intrinsic asthma, extrinsic asthma ($n=10$) and controls ($n=14$). Mean ± SE

	Recovery (%)	Total cells	Macrophages (%)	Lymphocytes (%)	Neutrophils (%)	Eosinophils (%)
Extrinsic asthma	38±4.0	12.2±3.9	79±4.0	10±4.1	3±0.5	8±2.7
Intrinsic asthma	28±3.4	12.7±2.6	63±5.8	14±3.4	15±5.5	8±2.9
Controls	39±3.6	11.7±1.9	86±2.5	8±1.5	4±1	2±0.5

These results agree in part with the findings of Tomioka et al. (1984) who also found an increased percentage of mast cells in the bronchoalveolar lavage of asthmatic subjects. However, the percentage of mast cells in both asthmatics and controls was lower in their study than in the one reported here and there was no significant difference between asthmatics and controls with respect to the histamine content of the lavage. This difference is likely to be due to differences in lavage technique and the subsequent processing of bronchoalveolar cells as discussed in Chap. 3. This group used a smaller lavage volume, filtered recovered fluid and cells through gauze, stained in suspension rather than on cytocentrifuge smears and used different fixatives. Minor differences in technique between laboratories may result in large differences in results (Mordelet-Dambrine et al. 1984).

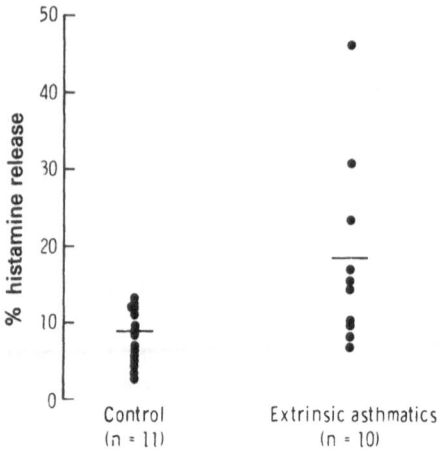

Fig. 7.2.   Spontaneous release of histamine from BAL mast cells.

There are several functional differences between bronchoalveolar mast cells from subjects with extrinsic asthma and controls. Asthmatic bronchoalveolar mast cells appear to be less stable in vitro with an increase in the spontaneous release of histamine during the course of a 10 min incubation at 37°C (Fig. 7.2); this release was widely variable (7.1%–46.5%) and tended to be greatest in those subjects with asthma of greatest clinical severity. This high spontaneous release may be related to the trauma implicit in the way in which these cells are obtained rather than being indicative of an ongoing in vivo phenomenon. Nevertheless, spontaneous release from cells of control subjects is much less, which would suggest an inherent instability of bronchoalveolar mast cells from asthmatic subjects. It is interesting to speculate that this instability may be involved in the pathogenesis of bronchoconstriction induced by non-immunological mechanisms. For example, exercise-induced bronchoconstriction has been related to respiratory heat exchange (Deal et al. 1979); therefore one factor that may be involved in the increased spontaneous release of histamine observed in vitro may be the cooling of these cells from 37°C down to 20°C during the lavage procedure.

Immunological activation of bronchoalveolar mast cells from subjects with extrinsic asthma by anti-IgE (Fig. 7.3) or allergen (Fig. 7.4) to which the patient is sensitive results in histamine release. In the case of anti-IgE, this release was significantly accentuated when compared with controls, an increased proportion

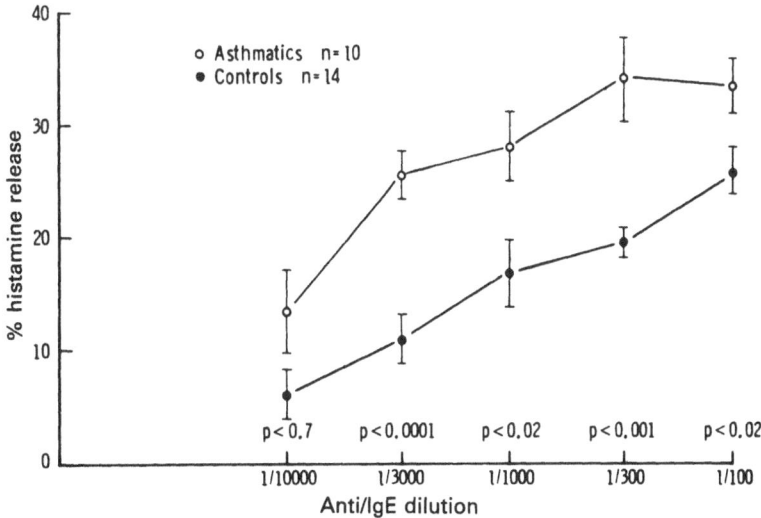

Fig. 7.3. Anti-IgE induced histamine release from bronchoalveolar cells of extrinsic asthmatics ($n=10$) and controls ($n=14$). *Points* represent means with SE bars.

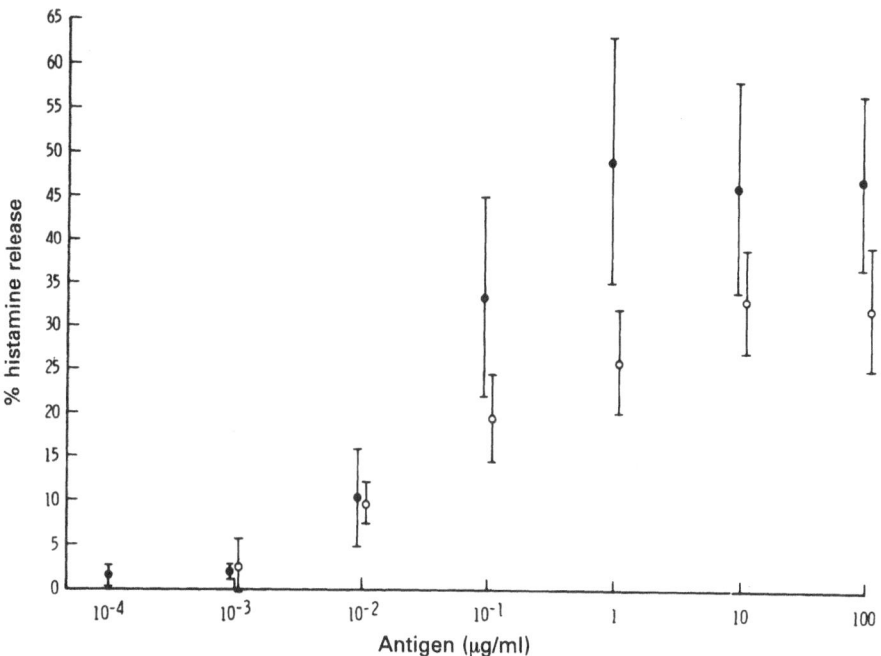

Fig. 7.4. Antigen induced histamine release from peripheral blood leucocytes (●) and broncho-alveolar cells (○) of subjects with extrinsic asthma (house dust mite antigen $n=7$, grass pollen $n=1$).

of cellular histamine being released at all effective dilutions of anti-IgE. This accentuation of release appeared to be confined to the lung, for despite differences in serum IgE between the two groups, IgE-dependent histamine release from peripheral basophils was similar in both asthmatics and controls (Fig. 7.5). Findlay and Lichtenstein (1980) have also reported no differences in anti-IgE induced histamine release from basophils of asthmatics and controls. The increased responsiveness of bronchoalveolar mast cells to IgE-dependent stimulus may reflect increased local concentrations of IgE or an alteration in IgE receptor-response coupling. Further investigation is required to distinguish these possibilities.

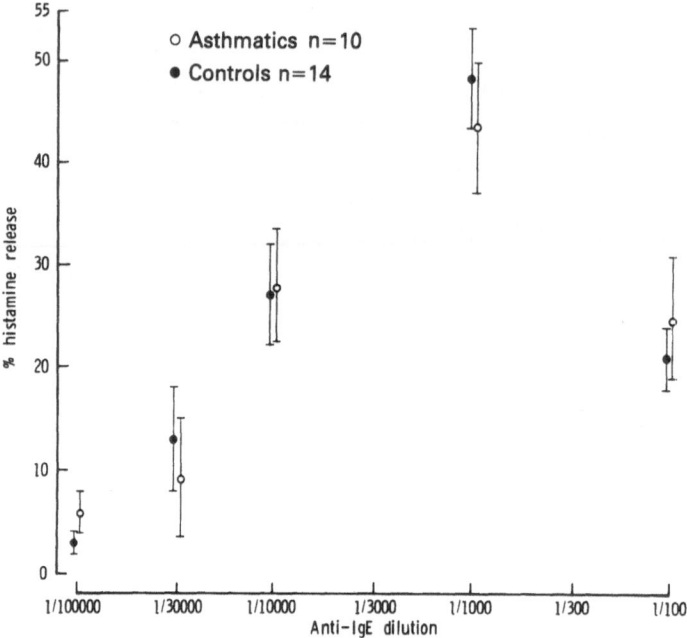

Fig. 7.5. Anti-IgE induced histamine release from peripheral blood leucocytes of asthmatic subjects ($n=10$) and controls ($n=14$). *Points* represent means with SE bars.

Challenge with specific allergen (grass pollen or house dust mite) resulted in histamine release in a dose-dependent fashion from bronchoalveolar mast cells and peripheral blood basophils of asthmatic subjects, but not from non-atopic controls. Antigens (allergens) which are normally inhaled therefore have the capacity to cause mediator release from sensitised mast cells lying superficially within the lungs of subjects with extrinsic asthma.

Intrinsic Asthma

The situation in intrinsic asthma is less clear. Fewer subjects with late onset, skin test negative, reversible airflow obstruction have been studied and some were on

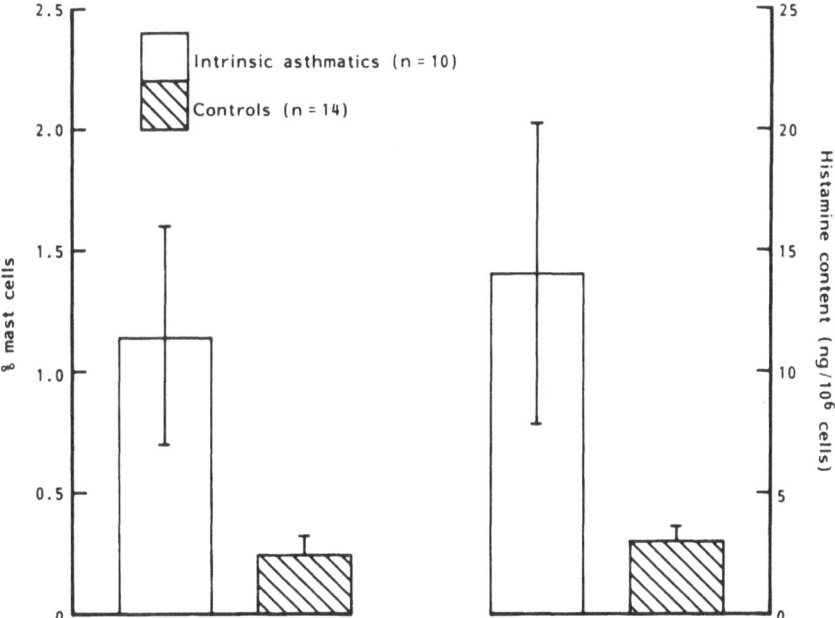

Fig. 7.6. Histogram showing difference between control subjects and patients with intrinsic asthma for percent of mast cells recovered by bronchoalveolar lavage and the histamine content of these cells.

regular steroid therapy. As the effects of steroid therapy on the bronchoalveolar cell population are unknown, interpretation of the results available in the subjects with intrinsic asthma who underwent BAL is difficult. However, both the percentage of mast cells and the histamine content of the bronchoalveolar cell population were significantly increased in subjects with intrinsic asthma when compared with controls ($P<0.01$; Fig. 7.6). This difference was present both in five subjects on oral or high dose inhaled steroids and five subjects on low dose inhaled beclomethasone (200 μg/day) or on no steroid therapy at all. Thus an increased percentage of mast cells in bronchoalveolar lavage is a feature of both intrinsic and extrinsic asthma. In addition, the percentage of neutrophils and the percentage of eosinophils were increased in the lavage of subjects with intrinsic asthma (Table 7.2).

Bronchoalveolar cells from both extrinsic and intrinsic asthmatics also have certain functional characteristics in common. The spontaneous release of histamine from bronchoalveolar mast cells of intrinsic asthmatics is significantly greater than from those of controls ($P<0.01$). In addition, although dose-response curves were available for only four subjects not currently taking oral or high dose corticosteroids, there appears to be an accentuation of IgE-dependent histamine release with respect to controls in much the same way as in subjects

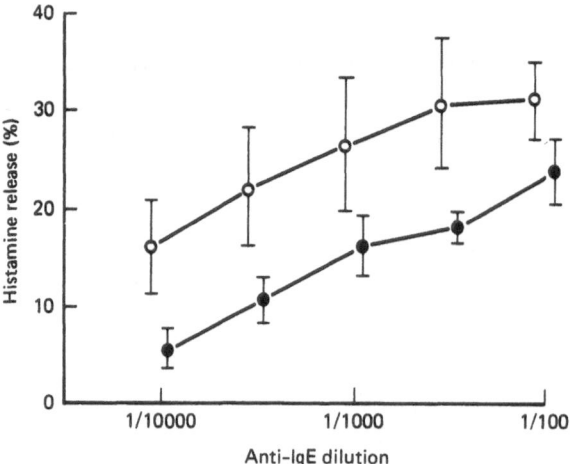

Fig. 7.7. Anti-IgE induced histamine release from subjects with intrinsic asthma ($n=4$, ○) compared with controls ($n=14$, ●). *Points* represent means with SE bars.

with extrinsic asthma (Fig. 7.7). Challenge with house dust mite antigen did not lead to histamine release from the bronchoalveolar cells of the three subjects with intrinsic asthma in which it was tested.

These common abnormalities of bronchoalveolar mast cell number and function in subjects with intrinsic or extrinsic asthma are of particular interest. The aetiology of intrinsic asthma remains obscure. The observations here might suggest a common pathogenesis for the two conditions. Increased numbers of specifically sensitised mast cells within the airways of subjects with extrinsic asthma may explain their rapid response to inhaled antigen. An inherent instability of this population in subjects with both intrinsic and extrinsic asthma may also explain the bronchoconstrictor response to non-immunological stimuli such as infection, water mist, sulphur dioxide, exercise and hyperventilation (mediated either by airway cooling or changes in osmolarity of lung lining fluid). This latter possibility would be in keeping with the finding that sodium cromoglycate protects against such non-specific stimuli, without effect on histamine or methacholine reactivity (Patel 1984).

Antigen challenge in by far the majority of cases will occur via the airways. Lying superficially within these airways, bronchoalveolar mast cells would be in an ideal position to interact with such inhaled antigen and mediators released by bronchoalveolar mast cells would immediately be in direct contact with the airway surface. Bronchoalveolar mast cells would therefore be ideally placed to mediate the rapid bronchial reactions which follow the inhalation of allergen in asthmatic subjects. There is therefore the potential for antigen-specific mediator release from mast cells lying superficially within lungs of subjects with asthma.

The consequences of mediator release from mast cells lying superficially within the airway mucosa or on the airway surface are speculative. After the initial interaction between mast cell and antigen at or near the airway surface, amplification of the response may occur in several ways. Mast cell mediators may recruit secondary cells such as alveolar macrophages or submucosal mast cells into the reaction with further release of inflammatory and bronchoconstrictor mediators. An alternative route by which the effect of degranulation of superficial mast cells may be amplified is by the action of mast cell mediators on local nerve endings causing reflex bronchoconstriction. The effects of mast cell mediators on mucosal permeability may also be important, with interruption of tight junctions allowing the penetration of antigen to the numerous mast cells in the airway submucosa. Finally, released mediators would have a direct effect on airway smooth muscle, mucus glands, goblet cells and vascular permeability. None of these effects are mutually exclusive and all may play a part in the events that follow antigen inhalation, or non-immunological challenge of subjects with asthma.

Effect of Corticosteroids

Despite their therapeutic use in bronchial asthma for many years, the mode of action of corticosteroids remains unclear. An attempt was therefore made to analyse the findings of bronchoalveolar lavage in these asthmatic subjects in terms of the presence or absence of steroid therapy. Unfortunately, the two groups, those currently on oral or high dose inhaled therapy and those on only low dose inhaled beclomethasone or no steroid therapy, were poorly matched. There were more subjects in the non-steroid treated group ($n=13$) than the steroid treated group ($n=7$) and more of the former were extrinsic asthmatics whereas the majority of the latter were intrinsic asthmatics. The results must therefore be interpreted with great caution. Nevertheless, whilst there was no apparent difference between these groups with respect to mast cell percentages, histamine content and spontaneous histamine release, the IgE-dependent release of histamine was depressed in the steroid treated group. This was noted both in the group of asthmatics as a whole and also in the intrinsic asthmatics only ($n=4$ oral or high dose inhaled steroids, $n=4$ low dose inhaled steroids or no steroid). This finding might appear contradictory to reports suggesting that although corticosteroids inhibit the late response to antigen challenge in vivo, they have no effect on the immediate asthmatic reaction. However, there is now evidence to show that prolonged treatment with corticosteroids in vivo causes a reduction to both the early and the late response to bronchial provocation with antigen. The degree of inhibition of the immediate response by corticosteroids on treatment in vivo increases from 1 to 4 weeks (Dahl and Johansson 1982). All of our steroid treated subjects had been on oral or high dose inhaled corticosteroids for a minimum of 2 weeks. Furthermore one week's pretreatment with inhaled budesonide will lead to a reduction in the release of histamine in response to nasal allergen challenge in subjects with allergic rhinitis (Pipkorn and Andersson 1982). In preliminary experiments in vitro, preincubation of human bronchoalveolar or dispersed lung mast cells with either betamethasone or dexamethasone, failed to inhibit the IgE-dependent release of histamine (unpublished observations). Nevertheless, one possible mode of action of corticosteroids after prolonged use in vivo may be to reduce the release of mast cell mediators, a possibility that requires further investigation. In support of this hypothesis it has recently been shown that steroids down-regulate IgE receptors or mast cells in vitro; also decreased mediator release is observed (Bergstrand et al. 1986).

References

Bergstrand H, Lundquist B, Paterson BA (1986) The glucocorticosteroid budesonide partially blocks histamine release from human lung tissue in vitro. Allergy 41: 319–326

Dahl R, Johansson SA (1982) Importance of duration of treatment with inhaled budesonide on the immediate and late bronchial reaction. Eur J Resp Dis 63 (Suppl 122): 167–175

Deal EC, McFadden ER, Ingram RH, Strauss RH, Jaeger JJ (1979) Role of respiratory heat exchange in the production of exercise-induced asthma. J Appl Physiol 46: 467–475

Diaz P, Galleguillos FR, Gonzales MC, Pantin CFA, Kay AB (1984) Bronchoalveolar lavage in asthma: the effect of disodium cromoglycate on leucocyte counts, immunoglobulins and complement. J Allergy Clin Immunol 74: 41–48

Findlay SR, Lichtenstein LM (1980) Basophil releasability in patients with asthma. Am Rev Resp Dis 122: 53–59

Flint KC, Leung KBP, Hudspith BN, Brostoff J, Pearce FL, Johnson NMcI (1985) Bronchoalveolar mast cells in extrinsic asthma: a mechanism for the initiation of antigen specific bronchoconstriction. Br Med J 291: 923–926

Goddard P, Chantreuil J, Damon M, Coupe M, Flandre O, Paulet AC, Michel FB (1982) Functional assessment of alveolar macrophages: comparison of cells from asthmatic and normal subjects. J Allergy Clin Immunol 70: 88–93

Joseph M, Tonnel AB, Torpier G, Capron A, Arnoux B, Bienveniste J (1983) Involvement of immunoglobulin E in the secretory process of alveolar macrophages from asthmatic patients. J Clin Invest 71: 221–230

Mordelet-Dambrine M, Arnoux A, Stanislas-Le Guern G, Sandron D, Chretien J, Huchon G (1984) Processing of lung lavage fluid causes variability in the bronchoalveolar cell count. Am Rev Resp Dis 130: 305–306

National Heart, Lung and Blood Institute Workshop (1985) Summary and recommendations of a workshop on the investigative use of fibreoptic bronchoscopy and bronchoalveolar lavage in asthmatics. Am Rev Resp Dis 132: 180–182

Patel KR (1984) Sodium cromoglycate and bronchial reactivity. Clin Allergy 14: 143–145

Pipkorn B, Andersson U (1982) Budesonide and nasal mucosal histamine content and anti-IgE induced histamine release. Allergy 37: 591–595

Tomioka M, Ida S, Shindoh Y, Ishihara T, Takishima T (1984) Mast cells in the bronchoalveolar lumen of patients with bronchial asthma. Am Rev Resp Dis 129: 1000–1005

Subject Index